T0245852

WOMEN ARE ANGRY

WOMEN ARE ANGRY

WHY YOUR RAGE IS HIDING AND HOW TO LET IT OUT

JENNIFER COX

First published in the UK by Lagom
An imprint of the Zaffre Publishing Group
A Bonnier Books UK Company
4th Floor, Victoria House,
Bloomsbury Square,
London, WC1B 4DA

Owned by Bonnier Books
Sveavägen 56, Stockholm, Sweden

Hardback – 978-1-785120-93-0
Ebook – 978-1-785120-94-7
Audio – 978-1-785120-95-4

A CIP catalogue of this book is available from the British Library.

Designed and typeset by EnvyDesign Ltd
Printed and bound by Clays Ltd, Elcograf S.p.A

1 3 5 7 9 10 8 6 4 2

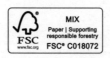

Every reasonable effort has been made to trace copyright holders of material
reproduced in this book, but if any have been inadvertently overlooked the
publishers would be glad to hear from them.

Lagom is an imprint of Bonnier Books UK
www.bonnierbooks.co.uk

To my women.
And of course, to my men. Who stand beside me,
and dream of better.

Contents

Introduction   1

Part One   THE SITUATION   7

Chapter One   **You're Being Gaslit**   9

Chapter Two   **What Anger Does to Our Bodies**   15

Chapter Three   **What We Can Do About It**   25

Part Two   OUR STORY, FROM CRADLE TO GRAVE   29

Chapter Four   **Girl Baby**   31

Chapter Five   **Little Girl**   51

Chapter Six   **Tween Girl**   77

Chapter Seven   **Teen Girl**   101

Chapter Eight   **Young Woman**   129

Chapter Nine **Adult Woman**   165

Chapter Ten **Menopausal Woman**   205

Chapter Eleven **Older Woman**   231

Part Three The Solution   251

Chapter Twelve **Get It All Out**   253

Final Note: What Now?   277

Acknowledgements   287

Endnotes   289

AUTHOR'S NOTE

The case studies in this book are inspired by the many stories I'm told by women in my practice. I've amalgamated them into a handful of fictitious patients, who bear ethnically ambiguous names and about whom I provide little information as to heritage. This is intentional. I work with a diverse group of women: across race, class, sexuality, education, maternal status, marital status and profession. Their stories are universal, though, and any of them could be you.

Introduction

I'M A THERAPIST, and I have something disturbing to tell you. Women are in trouble. An autoimmune condition ravages our bodies and minds. I witness the devastation daily. The symptoms vary – from obsessive compulsive disorder (OCD) to anxiety, from migraine to depression to eczema. And there's a common cause: anger. Anger is eating us up, from the inside out. The pressures heaped on women by every level of society, and its systems, leave us furious. But we've been conditioned not to recognise our rage, so it burns behind the scenes. And, from there, it's destroying us.

Coming of age in dreamy nineties Britain, I was taught we'd largely outwitted the insidious harm of sexist constraint. In an age rendered glorious by corduroy, androgynous haircuts, Britpop and pickled sharks, tedious old misogyny was harder to spot. But it turns out it was there all along; it hadn't gone anywhere. How can we have mistaken the unregulated frontiers of ladette culture for some kind of ironic post-misogynist utopia? Silly us.

The most flagrant women-haters of today, preaching their overt messages of violence to a new generation of millions, alert us to the magnitude of women hatred worldwide. They also serve as a distraction; permitting that stealthier, time-worn brand of misogyny to slide in unseen. As in any other decade (just like the misguided nineties), covert acts of sexism play out through the myriad micro-interactions of a woman's day. But, today, the rules are more sophisticated – and we've somehow been playing along.

Well, I've stopped playing along. In my consulting room, I employ theory informed by psychoanalysis and neuroscience to help individual women from across the world make sense of their suffering. In many ways, though, it's like I'm applying a Band-Aid to a haemorrhage. When an entire ecosystem is sick, we question the value of treating a single organism.

I have written this book as I want to provide us all with the means to challenge our individual agony, as well as to start a wider conversation about why the hell this is happening to us – and how we can make it stop.

To this end, I need to outline the reasons why an insidious, rather than overt, sexism has become baked into women's psyches and how our upbringing helps secure this own-goal. Partially, this is because we're told that sexism no longer exists; copious gender equality policies attest to that. But it's also because women are conditioned *not* to feel the most obvious signal for injustice: anger. So, when frustration or irritated confusion surface at some outmoded sexist incident, we don't accept that emotion at face value. Instead, we subdue it, shrug it off, explain it away – normally at deeply unconscious levels – and our bodies are left to make sense of what's happening.

Unfortunately, our poor bodies are pretty basic in this respect. They don't have a lot of nuanced options for expressing pain and suffering. Even our brains have few distinct pathways for communicating their turmoil. As a psychotherapist, I see the evidence in my practice daily. Women present feeling sad and anxious, or suffering from a range of somatic symptoms – from panic attacks to tension headaches, from irritable bowel syndrome (IBS) to eating disorders. Women are twice as likely as men to suffer depression, three times more likely to experience migraines and four times more likely to be diagnosed with autoimmune disease.

I've been scouring the history books for clues about the origin of this suffering. There seems to have been a global pivot away from sexual parity after agricultural economies began to dominate, as we shifted to a more sedentary way of life. Darwin himself had some choice views on sex differences and, indeed, promoted the finding that women were inferior in body and mind. He gave us 'natural selection': it turns out, he also laid the groundwork for the gender pay gap, limited reproductive rights and legal injustices.

But we can't leave it all at Darwin's door. There have been countless opportunities to address these issues, since the word 'sexism' was immortalised by the US feminist Caroline Bird Mahoney more than half a century ago in her speech, 'On Being Born Female'. Real change just seems to elude us. From before we are born, we're saddled with society's projections and expectations, which eventually begin to distort us at a near-cellular level. We come into the world knowing what's expected;

it's woven into the soft fabric of our psyche. Even the word 'sexism' feels so beige now, so overused – and yet also weirdly underused. It loses meaning and feels alienating. I even feel a bit *embarrassed* writing it now. Can't we come up with a jazzier version? A 'sexism' for our time? Something which conveys the nimbleness of the patriarchy, the way it consistently remains one step ahead …

In my London clinic, I work with women from across diverse demographics. I'm witness to the constant reinforcing interplay of 'sexist' social structures and its various family-specific permutations, handed down through generations like an ugly old wardrobe that belonged to our gran and is somehow too massive and unwieldy for anyone to ditch. It just carries on sitting there and we form all sorts of narratives around it, to do with guilt and tradition. We may all hate it, but it seems we're stuck with it. Our parents, too, were born within the shadow of these structures. As their parents before them, they operate within this creaking edifice, and become the unconscious harbingers of our destiny. Statements like, 'A son is a son until he finds him a wife; a daughter is yours for the rest of her life' go deep. We just *know* this stuff – we know what's expected of us without being told. But we know it at such a deep level that we don't even notice that we know it.

Our capacity to question is ambushed by our lack of confidence: something feels wrong, but we can't conceive what it could be. I'm talking about *good girl* expectations: about doing what you're told, putting others first, excusing people's bad behaviour, feeling as if certain school subjects are more *your* subjects. I'm talking about the sense that it would be impolite to say *no* to someone, or not do something, simply because you

4

don't want to. I'm talking about always feeling you're in the wrong; an instinct that *you* should apologise. That if you aren't comfortable with something, it's your problem. When you've been told across generations that things just *are* a certain way, it's practically impossible to crawl out from under that. So we sink. We internalise.

Contemporary medicine prescribes pills which, sadly, are blunt instruments when it comes to treating psychological pain. When our own brains are incapable of distinguishing between states of rage and states of depression, pity the health professional attempting to help decipher the difference. As women, we're still a long way from being able to recognise our own anger.

I urge us to get to work immediately on identifying both the rage and its causes, in order to avoid detrimental health outcomes. Much of our individual anger ultimately seems to stem from trying to be a woman in a world which still makes life very difficult for women. A *patriarchal* world; a world where history, geography, privilege and structure have been dominated by men. Through the identification of repeated themes shared by numerous international patients of all ages, I want to help you tune in to your own feelings of frustration and impotent rage.

The scientific underpinning of why anger is so damaging if left unrecognised is key to how I suggest we treat the disease. As the case studies woven through this book reveal, our approach needs to focus on physical and expressive forms of release. The remarkable impact on lives and health when we finally tap into our rage should be everyone's privilege. But our first task is to understand the cause. Our anger comes from the gaslighting we've grown up with, the pretence that we're living in a world which has changed for the better.

Part One

THE SITUATION

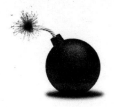

CHAPTER ONE

You're Being Gaslit

WE'RE SUFFERING, BUT we've become so used to the symptoms of our illness that we don't think about the cause anymore. We may have *never* actually thought about the cause, since the symptoms seem to have a validity of their own. Fibromyalgia (a condition that causes widespread pain and tiredness), postnatal depression (PND) and migraine are convincing diagnoses in their own right, aren't they? We accept them as the ordinary burden of our womanhood. What if they don't have to be? What if our suffering shuts us up, and prevents us from asking questions about *why* things need to be experienced so violently in our own bodies?

There's a shared incentive to this group denial. If the gender equality policies intended to scramble the power imbalance don't work, perhaps nothing will. The reality is too unbearable to consider. Thus, we turn away and fail to consider it. We pretend it can't be real; we look at all the ways instead that women *seem* to be able to Have It All, though, admittedly, our bodies are breaking and, in many cases, so are our minds. The 'solutions' are abundant: Get ye to a yoga retreat! Take an antidepressant! It's because you're not fasting for long enough!

This is collaborative gaslighting on a massive scale – and gaslighting makes people feel angry. Its correct usage denotes the way a mind can be manipulated so that its sense of reality is damaged. This wound is what I hear described in the consulting room every day: the realities of women's *actual* lives, not the imagined versions they tell themselves they desired and so must somehow be having. This double deception of *not having* something we need and living with the consequences of that (whilst simultaneously being told that we *do* have it) is a conflict which we must ultimately house within us. We have to house it within us because nobody's offering to take it from us. We need this conversation to change direction.

So, it's starting now. Here.

Together, we're going to learn to identify our feelings of rage, understand what they're trying to tell us, figure out a shared language for expressing it and get talking. But this isn't just the woman's job; this isn't about allocating her more work.

Men, come in and join our party! Please understand that we're talking about a *system*. The one most easily referred to as 'patriarchy', in which you've also grown up. The one which has us all by the scruff of the neck. The one that wanted us, the women, to figure out how to Have It All, but didn't extend the same challenge to men.

You might indeed wish very much to share 'the load' with women, but your work doesn't give you realistic parenting leave, you're eyed with suspicion if you're the only dad at a kids' party, and your school sent boys out of the classroom when it was time to talk about 'periods', so you still feel a bit confused about how they work. We know you're angry too – the patriarchy hardly makes it easy for you. Here, though, we're talking about the people who have, historically, been prohibited from showing their rage. Please know that this book isn't some resentful, dead-end accusation. This problem needs to be *our* problem. I'm asking you to stand with us; your sisters, girlfriends, wives and mums. Help us figure out what to do. Because *this* – what's happening now – is literally killing us.

Likewise, I need to ask women as they read this to drop the defence. Stop protecting people. The women I'm going to tell you about in this book didn't arrive in therapy using words like 'hate' and 'rage' and 'disgust'. They came in telling me they loved their family 'to bits' and were their mum's 'best friend'. But I want you to allow yourself to feel the real stuff whilst you're here with me. Let yourself feel the stuff that's been banging on the door of your unconscious. Let the real you breathe. Let her try out this powerful, gutsy vocabulary. Just like the women in this book now have.

The relief we feel when we shed the sexist blinkers and realise we're not losing our minds is visceral. I watch an increasing number of women understand that, actually, something systemically oppressive has grown in power in tandem with ourselves. Our mothers' and grandmothers' fight has undeniably awarded us privileges. We do undoubtedly hold more sway. But, as the beast within develops and evolves, so too must the fortress which contains it. Is it weird that I'm analogising women's growing power as a beast? Women's power is frightening to the patriarchy. It just is. It's an unknown force which could, in theory, knock men from their comfortable seat. It's pretty disturbing and bestial. It's witchy. Therefore, new ways of oppressing must be designed, in order to keep women limited. We're too dangerous as a force.

For their part, women may well concede they have more of a presence in the arenas they've chosen for themselves. But the experiences they have in these fields seem equally to highlight a sense of disempowerment, shutdown and inequity – quite contrary to the messaging around equality we've grown up expecting, and keep being told we've achieved.

What the hell is going on?

The women patients I see are initially confused – because they'd believed the gaslighting. They'd hoped so hard for change that they had to believe in the deception. Give them some subsidised childcare! That'll make it look as if we want them back at work (though costs still mean most women are *at best* breaking even during those early years of child-rearing). Commonly now, we're actually *losing* money to retain our careers until children go to school. And, even then, what about the holidays? What about the 3pm finish time? The gender pay gap widens further still when we add in the cost of childcare, which often comes straight out of a woman's pay packet, as the bill kicks off in tandem with her return to earning.

What about working hours? Let them work 'part-time'! (We won't pay them for the inevitable day and a half they work unseen, for fear we'll sack them if they don't.) We don't discriminate against mothers!

On the contrary, I give you my many female patients who find themselves demoted after maternity leave or, worse still, walking back into a watertight redundancy 'offer', or out-and-out sacking. Indeed, recent data from the campaign Pregnant Then Screwed found that 52 per cent of women face discrimination during their pregnancy, maternity leave or on return to work.

Society pretends that it's making allowances, that it's supportive, that it *gets* the issues and is responding to them. When I hear women tell me that they can't make a request or a complaint because people have already made so many allowances for them, I want to cry. It sounds so devastatingly like wide-scale fabrication. Very professional, polite abuse – but precedent-setting, nonetheless.

The aggregate effect of many such, apparently isolated, experiences eventually takes its toll. This book is dedicated to the resulting phenomenon I've seen burning through women over the past decade. Anger. A feverish, unstoppable rage buried beneath a plethora of symptoms, both psychological and physical, which are called all manner of things, from anxiety to PND, which are obviously both valid diagnoses. But lazy labelling can prevent deeper questions. Doctors are taught to listen to the patient, that 'the patient will tell you'. These patients *are* telling them. But they haven't been listening.

In my role as a psychotherapist, I'm trying to correct this. I *have* been listening, and what I bring you is a set of themes I hear repeated daily, of how this anger is making women ill and that it stems from the systems which surround us and clamp themselves to us from before the day we're born.

Our anger doesn't present very often in its straightforward form. It's disguised psychologically as panic attacks or OCD, and very often physiologically through chronic pain or migraine or fatigue. It is *displaced* anger. Other emotions come in like an apparently sheltering wall – sadness, tearfulness, shame, numbness, guilt. They push the original rage out of the way and sit more easily in our minds and within the role that society has carved out for us. And, when we dig down, a lot of the anger seems to stem from trying to navigate a world set up for and by men. Confronted with the seeming impossibility of that *ever* changing, we're left to do our best to handle the oceans of unbearable rage, which ultimately feel so intolerable that we need to repress them, just to get on with another contradictory day. This territory is not untrodden. The incredible work of trauma expert Gabor Maté and psychiatrist Bessel van der Kolk has also identified the connection between mind and body, stress and illness. But what I've seen in women requires an expansion of these ideas. I believe that the structures of society itself contribute to the architecture of our ill health. I believe that properly expressing our feelings about what is happening to us at a societal and family level will ultimately help to heal us.

Expressing needs to be the opposite of repressing. Instinctively, we know this to be true. And it's exactly those pre-socially conditioned instincts we need to get back to. We need to tune in, and transfer excess negative energy outwards. Through talking, yes, but, when words just aren't enough or we can't find them yet, through that self-same physicality which senses and stores these uncomfortable feelings. Sometimes, a little bit of outwardly-directed, forceful energy release is exactly what the doctor ordered, especially when what we're up against is vast volumes of generational and societal gaslighting. We wear that kind of trauma on the inside. The pent-up, self-harming rage this induces needs to be expelled before we can take control.

CHAPTER TWO

What Anger Does to Our Bodies

THOUSANDS OF YEARS of ancestral evolution have anchored anger into our psychological repertoire. Just as any nature documentary featuring gorillas bears out, anger (one of the five 'basic emotions') is critical for hierarchical organisation, reproduction and sustenance. The motivation is the same at a human level. Anger can be pro-social. It enables us to impose structure, defend supplies and calculate threat. It can be a force for our real benefit, when we harness it. Put in very basic terms, anger is decided in our brain's reward circuitry. When there's a disparity between our expectation and reality, between what we were envisaging as a 'reward' and that being somehow thwarted, our amygdala (the brain region chiefly concerned with emotional processes) is alerted and feelings of anger flow. The behaviour which follows is moderated by our prefrontal cortex, which is really only fully formed in our late twenties, and is our kind of behavioural office manager.

When we talk about anger, we're actually talking about a multiverse of feeling. 'Anger' encompasses myriad emotions – from suppressed aggression to outward violence, from frustration or impotent helplessness to a sense of hurt, bitterness or loss; grievance about events experienced as unjust, people we feel have wounded us and experiences which have left us humiliated, exploited, manipulated or crushed …

The chemistry behind 'angry' states of mind is shared by moods more conventionally seen as depressive or anxious. Whilst in depression, anger is inverted and hidden, we can see the similarity more clearly with symptoms of anxiety. From phobia to social anxiety to overthinking, we observe elevated heart rate, sweating and shallow breathing. An angry body demonstrates these same hallmarks. This is no surprise when you recall that both have the 'stress' hormones adrenaline and cortisol at their chemical core. Psychologists Stanley Schachter and Jerome Singer were key players in helping to illustrate the extent to which the *interpretation* of our emotions is key to our experience. In an influential experiment in 1962, they detailed the way in which participants told two different narratives following an adrenaline shot. One group experienced 'euphoria' and the other 'anger'. This experiment alone evidences the need to start thinking about states of arousal in a different way: could we call anxiety 'excitement', given the right circumstances, for example?

Inflammation is the physical explanation shared by both anger and depression, and is currently my favourite candidate for the very similar symptoms exhibited by both. Anger has been linked to inflammation; specifically with elevated blood levels of the inflammatory markers c-reactive protein and cytokines, such as interleukin-6. Numerous meta-analyses find that the levels of those same acute-phase proteins and pro-inflammatory cytokines are elevated in patients with major depression.

Let's consider the ordinary role of inflammation. It occurs when chemical mediators produced by the body's white blood cells enter the bloodstream and tissues. The immediate release of chemicals, from histamine to prostaglandin, forms a defending army, aimed to protect the body from viral or bacterial invasion. Damaged tissue sends its own chemical signals, to which white blood cells respond by releasing compounds prompting cellular division and tissue regrowth. The inflammatory process can be acute (disappearing within hours) or chronic (lasting for months or even years). Conditions associated with chronic inflammation range from cancer to Alzheimer's disease. In autoimmune diseases like arthritis, the immune system triggers inflammation unnecessarily, causing damage as it fights regular tissues as if they are infected or diseased.

Although inflammation is a typical physiological response, required to enable the healing of injured tissue, in chronic cases the process fails to end once the wound has healed. It might even begin when no injury has been incurred. Chronic inflammation might follow infections that don't clear up or atypical immune reactions to healthy tissue. But longer-term elevations in inflammation have also been linked to the experience of chronic feelings of anger. Over time, increased levels of inflammation can impact our cell DNA, and have been linked to diseases like diabetes and cancer, and even to obesity.

The bidirectional relationship of depression with auto-immune disease is firmly established, meaning that people with these diseases – from multiple sclerosis (MS) and autoimmune thyroiditis to IBS – are also likely to report major depression. But, crucially, people with depression are at increased likelihood of reporting autoimmune disease. The brain seems to hurt along with the body – and vice versa.

You can see the associations here. Anger and depression have shared chemical substrates. Both states of mind also seem to co-occur with inflammation, and repressed anger can function in part as a predisposing factor. Interestingly for us, the impact of early life trauma on inflammation is observed in patients with major depression. Many researchers argue for the wealth of clinical and pre-clinical evidence that negative childhood events result in an ongoing elevation of inflammation. The picture is clear, although the language of science still seems to keep anger and depression apart when identifying their compatible relationship with inflammation. This needs to be addressed. An injured brain triggers inflammation. Likewise, inflammation in the body results in psychological pain. Just as pain in the body and pain in the mind are two sides of the same coin, anger and depression are too.

The physiology is too simple; the root cause is so much more complex. A diagnosis amounts to a shutdown. 'Anxiety' becomes the 'hysteria' of our day, a tool with which to stifle and suppress. And labels, diagnoses and pills become the asylum. 'Brand them with ME or IBS or OCD and throw away the key …'

This wraparound relationship between mind and body, anger and pain is told in diverse everyday conditions we, as women, frequently present with. An inner-city GP with whom I work closely has long remarked on the way in which women internalise and somatise their feeling. For example, we store anger in our muscles, often experienced as aches and tension.

WHAT ANGER DOES TO OUR BODIES

Surface electromyography (which measures muscle activation) indicates recruitment of muscles across our upper arms and shoulders in tandem with the experience of angry emotion. What happens when we don't end up hitting out or pushing away or exiting the situation like a springbok? What happens when this feeling simply sits, unrecognised, just hanging about in our bodies? When the tension finds an uncomfortable reservoir in our jaw, neck or shoulders, we know that headaches regularly follow. Studies have zoned in on the association between migraine and problems with the expression of anger, but more on that later.

And what about our other organs? What's going on there, hidden away, sparked by our equally packed-down and covert furious feelings? Across global institutions involved in biobehavioural health research, studies repeatedly demonstrate the impact and connections of psychological stress on our bodies – often by way of inflammatory markers. Time and again, they provide the clinical evidence for what I'm witnessing on the frontline.

Take your heart, for example. When your heart rate and blood pressure elevate, which happens as a response to anger, the possibility of hypertension creeps in. This is when the pressure in your blood vessels is too great. Pop! The stress hormones associated with anger (cortisol and adrenaline) create an increase in levels of sugar and fatty acid in the bloodstream. This contributes to the build-up of arterial plaque, and scratches away at our blood vessels. All in, remaining in sustained states of suppressed anger can increase the likelihood of stroke, Type 2 diabetes, cardiovascular diseases and heart attacks. Not great. But I haven't yet touched on your poor lungs ... Brace yourself.

Elevated hostility levels have been associated with worse baseline lung function readings and, across time, an accelerated reduction in lung function, regardless of any smoking. Again, scientists posit inflammation as the physical outcome of these higher hostility scores. As we're beginning to learn, elevated inflammation readings are physically destructive. In this case, they can increase our risk of pulmonary disease.

Because pain and anger are controlled by the same parts of our brains, you possibly won't be surprised to read that researchers connect the two experiences in other ways. The same areas of our cortex light up like beacons in functional magnetic resonance imaging (fMRI) studies exploring social rejection and emotional hurt as do with physical pain. A single, economical evolutionary pathway seems to have emerged which alerts us to both physical and emotional suffering. The experience of fibromyalgia, myalgic encephalomyelitis (ME, also called chronic fatigue syndrome) or atypical facial pain can be disabling, and often feel unbearable for the sufferer. This category of chronic, 'nociplastic pain' describes non-specific pain which is unconnected to an obvious cause, such as tissue damage. Although these conditions are complex, and I wouldn't suggest they can all straightforwardly be entirely answered by the solution of repressed rage, I do think we need to look carefully at the potential relationship. Research shows that the part of our brain involved in communicating nociplastic pain is actually concerned with regulating emotion. If you're unfortunate enough to suffer with enduring non-explained back pain, for example, you might notice that the condition worsens with anger. Researchers have noticed that sensations of physical pain can actually be incited by strong negative emotion. Additionally, increased inflammation leads to greater levels of pain. I hope you're beginning to see the entanglement of squashed down, undealt-with anger, and the strain it exerts on our poor bodies ...

When society places such a blanket ban on the expression of a certain feeling in half of its population, and when science clearly points to an association between difficulties expressing negative emotion with poor pronounced physical outcome, we'd be daft not to listen.

Our bodies are *really trying* to get us to do just that. They know something's up. Certain things we readily accept – the fact that, when we're nervous or anxious, we can feel nauseous, for example. But do we allow our bodies to tell us the full story? Or do we just move on once we feel better, and try to forget it happened? Listen up! Let it speak! The gut (comprised of your stomach and both intestines) houses its own nervous system, known as the enteric system, a constituent of the autonomic nervous system (ANS). This separate system can actually operate independently of your brain, with more neurons than the whole of the spinal cord (in the region of 400–600 million). The enteric nervous system comprises swathes of neurons, snuggled into the roughly 9 metres of our gut wall. Those neurons control both motor and sensory functions of the gut itself and the contractions involved in the digestive process.

The gut and brain enjoy a two-way dialogue (governed chiefly by the vagus nerve – the longest nerve of the ANS responsible for digestion, heart rate and breathing, amongst other bodily functions). So, if we regularly find ourselves in heightened emotional states, the brain can actually influence the contractions involved in digestion – meaning that gastric distress, diarrhoea and constipation are typical presenting problems of anger. Of course, they're also associated with the other ways that anger can manifest – namely, through 'stress' and 'anxiety'. Even if we're not aware that the pressures around us are elevating our psychological state, because that psychological state has become so normal to us, our gut knows. The vagal pathway shares information between our brain and gut via neurotransmitters and hormones (all, in turn, playing a critical role in sleep, stress, pain and mood regulation). You know when you sleep badly, sometimes your stomach can feel really upset? This is why. Everything is connected. Ulcers, IBS and gastroesophageal reflux and inflammatory bowel disease (IBD) are all potential outcomes of a disruption to this intimate relationship. Doesn't it feel mean? That you're feeling horrible anyway, because society's pushing all of its crap onto you, but, because you might not be expressing this awful feeling, it finds this other way – which ultimately hurts you more.

You'll now be familiar with the scientific recognition of our trillions of gut bacteria (the gut microbiome) and how vital these are to health. Our microbiome talks to our enteric nervous system, which eventually communicates with our central nervous system, which is made up of the brain and spinal cord. So, there's mounting evidence for this incredible gut garden and its derivatives having a significant influence on behaviour and mood. If this relationship is disrupted by suppressed anger which induces gut symptoms like IBS, these issues then feed back to our brains, and we're stuck in a loop. Hopefully you're now convinced of the importance of tuning in! Gut instinct is real. We need to protect this relationship.

Just as with reactivity in the gut, our skin can flare with

the emotional overload and inverted release of inflammatory elements like anger. Conditions like psoriasis, acne, rosacea or eczema are all susceptible to the impact of turbulent emotion. Certain studies discuss the prevalence of severe hives and psoriasis to the communication of anger. This isn't to draw a direct cause and effect to anger and skin conditions, but more to highlight the research noting the tendency for repression of strong negative feelings to result in inflammation cues, which can get told in various ways through our skin. This can also be influenced by your behaviours when angry. If, when you're agitated, you have a habit of picking or worrying at your face or skin, this will likely exacerbate any conditions beginning to surface. Your buried rage will impact other aspects of your lifestyle – from sleep to diet. If your sleep is disturbed, or your diet is full of sugar (a known inflammatory) because you're reaching for internal blankets to soothe away the rage, your skin will no doubt tell the tale. Typically, we attribute these experiences to 'stress'. I would argue that, just as excitement and anxiety might be so easily confused, as women we've been taught to accept our anger as 'stress', which seems to serve as convincing evidence that the problem emanates from inside of us, and that it's therefore *on us* to grapple with it. I argue the reverse: that for too long our bodies have been used as a dumping ground for that which society has failed to figure out. Enough is enough, women! What are we going to do about this?

CHAPTER THREE

What We Can Do About It

THERAPISTS SEE IT ALL. If you work across the demographic and across all of adulthood, if you've worked through the Covid-19 pandemic and through the mental health crisis that followed, with people struggling to get any kind of state provision, you've seen more than all.

Nowadays, because of online working, we're taken into households, we're taken into offices, we sit with people in cars or walk with them in parks. Much of my work is international, and my patients come from diverse backgrounds and cultures, work across various industries, have different sexual orientations and varying family and living situations. But it's the same stories I'm hearing, the same rage on repeat.

Though it kills me to admit it, I accept I can't singlehandedly rewrite the issues which still plague us at a systemic level. But, at an individual level, I can begin at the end and work my way backwards, rewinding through the pathways, unpicking symptom from cause and helping to separate out the issues so that women themselves can start to feel more confident about questioning the reality they're in. About identifying the gaslight, the deception. You'll see from reading about my patients that, once symptoms are better under control, we can more calmly invite the people in our lives to join us in making changes which benefit everybody, from partners to children to parents to friends. In this way, a butterfly effect can slowly start to shift the endemic expectations of a society that were embedded across millennia, but which we've really outgrown.

So now, I want to help *you*.

Making changes at a personal level really can help to move things at social and political levels. And this is how the good effects of psychotherapy, of helping our minds to heal, can influence the health of the collective mind. Awareness breeds awareness. Which breeds understanding. Which breeds change. It's my hunch that the very tools our oppression has bred into us are the tools which now best equip us for dominance. As women, we've learnt how to do an unreasonable number of things at once, expecting little respect. We've learnt how to watchfully wait. Behind the scenes, our power has grown. We really are the beast. It's just that, currently, the beast is chewing its own arm in distressed desperation.

If anger is the basis for women's ill health, we need to confront where it's coming from. Because the causes of our rage feel so impossible to correct, we often deny the feeling itself, using the internalised sexist rhetoric that we *aren't angry*: 'Angry? I've just come back from a mindfulness retreat!' Our self-talk is a brilliant own-goal which keeps us subdued. We silence ourselves.

This is because part of the continued undercover mechanism

of sexism dictates that women are still not allowed to be angry. Society still can't allow us a vocabulary to weave our rage around. If it did, sexism itself would have to take a bashing. We'd use our feelings to identify it and drive it out. Currently structured, each permits the other. Covert sexism prevents articulation of anger. No one wants an angry wife or daughter. No one wants to *be* an angry wife or daughter. And for as long as our anger is sublimated, sexism remains rife.

Let's now take a walk through our lives, from cradle to grave. Through the stories of the women I've supported, I want to help *you* see the forces at play – right from the beginning of your existence – which shape you in ways which seem unremarkable and 'natural'. I want to help you question them, to notice the impact they've had and are having on your mind and body. And to start to wonder whether there are ways of pushing back, doing things differently or downright demanding better.

Part Two

OUR STORY,
FROM CRADLE
TO GRAVE

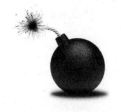

CHAPTER FOUR

Girl Baby

SINCE A WOMAN'S been taught to assume she's no longer facing discrimination in society, she's no longer on the lookout for it. This leads to an inability to identify and diagnose a lot of confused and ultimately angry feelings. The shocking part of this is that the die is cast before we're even born. 'You're expecting a Girl Baby? Fantastic! Someone to look after you when you're old' or 'You'll never be alone' or 'You'll be able to go shopping together!'

Or perhaps the more realistic response would be: 'You'll have to watch her try her hardest at every exam she ever sits, knowing that one day her brain will burst (literally) with the pressure of taking care of everybody else's emotional and physical needs, wondering at what point she should have stopped trying at school. Because at her job in the arts/in manufacturing/ on the shop floor/in banking, she is *definitely* being rewarded significantly less than the men who did worse than her through school!'

Or: 'Ooh? A Girl Baby! So you'll be looking forward to sitting with her through her development, as she feels disgusted by a body which seems to entrap her and have "Property of Society" stamped across it? Congrats!'

Who is Girl Baby, and what happens to someone burdened with a weight of impossible expectations, with a suitcase-load of *duty*, before she's even breathed air?

For starters, there's all the pink. Infants show clear colour preference by at least the age of 12 weeks. Because familiarity is such a huge driver in the formation of our tastes, if pink is endlessly flashed in front of you from even before this point, it's a no-brainer that this will become the locus towards which you gravitate. And pink is, indeed, still tenaciously flung at girls. Even the baby name cards issued at birth and stuck into the plastic hospital cots are pink. Go into any supermarket clothing aisle and you'll be flattened by variations on the theme; there's no mistaking what you're meant to buy for whom. This is just one of the wired-in social habits we're pretending has changed. And I know – it's so cute, I love it too! But are we just trained to love it? Men don't love it. They don't go – 'Ooh, get me some of that gorgeous pink winceyette mini sleep suit replete with bunny ears.' Well, if they do, they're pretty quiet about it …

As long as women carry and feed a baby, it seems impossible to achieve a genuine equality. This is a reality which doesn't get discussed. Rather, the pretence around it feeds the gaslighting. Lines of projection still mean we identify, if not merge, with our mothers. If the power of pink persists, even in families who have tried to curtail it, we should be realistic about other transferences. It's not the colour *per se* – it's what the colour represents; it's the associations and meanings that come riding along on its train.

If cars and trucks and dinosaurs and building blocks were also available in pink there'd be no issue. But we're instructed in feminised symbolism from this earliest point. Softness, cuteness, homeliness, pastel insipidity, infantilism, tweeness, *care*; every pink pyjama or glittery sandal or eraser says it. It reminds you of who you are, of what you're going to be drawn to. Humans will always gravitate towards what's familiar, even if it's not good for them, because our brains use less energy that way; it's their evolutionary MO.

Let's think about how girls' minds begin to develop differently according to this influence and modelling, reinforced by family and society expectations. And, through our case studies, observe how this differential influences behaviour. The seeds of social silencing are planted and pollinate into a garden of repressed rage. From this earliest point, we're subtly coerced and co-opted into various roles within families, couples, friendships and places of work. Let's explore – together – what we need to do to challenge this.

Here's an example of a patient whose tussle with the Girl Baby body she was born into left her scarred by a lifetime of warped pseudo-solutions. And who wanted to undo her experience by attempting to correct it in the subsequent generation.

Robin
Anger as migraine. Her strategy = The cold

Robin had just had her second baby – another boy – when she started coming to see me. She was distraught. 'I'd wanted a girl, I'd pictured a girl. And the awful thing is ... This is what Mum did with me!' Ironically, she'd been her own mother's un-chosen second girl. Her mum had visualised a boy, had been so confident she hadn't scanned, and really expected one to pop out.

Robin's family had been apparently progressive in its values (whatever that *really* means, when you consider the depth of our wiring. That massive, clunky wardrobe ...). Nonetheless, Robin's mum had been so desperate for her baby to be a boy that she'd already named him and started kitting out the 'nursery' with all things masculine.

'For people who were allegedly so right-on, they were surprisingly rigid in their view of gendered play things!' Robin realised. 'My mum had been so convinced that she'd even got my dad to buy a Lego construction set. They painted the nursery according to their view of boy theme, blah blah.' Robin rolled her eyes and looked disgusted. 'But listen to what happened next ...'

Robin had everything she needed physically. She was fed, taken to dance classes and lived in a nice house. But she was fundamentally unwanted. And she felt it. She may not have been able to control the fact that she hadn't been born a boy, but she was bright, and she recognised a solution. She could at least curry favour by being the *most girl*. Her mind began to adapt to the problem of being in this less-than body, representative of something so partial and disappointing. Robin didn't arrive with this narrative neatly sewn up. It took us a while to piece together the memories, the realisations, the understanding.

One fact she was certain of, though, was how she'd tried really hard to turn the system to her advantage, to call its bluff. Pink was almost laughably her calling card. Dirt was treated as an allergen. And then, Robin's little cousin, Callie, was born. The two were brought up in a tight-knit family. When Callie was diagnosed with learning difficulties, Robin stepped up. Now, she would finally be appreciated. Now she had worth. In her hyper-feminised solution state, she became the best listener, the prettiest, the most self-erasing, and translator of her cousin's needs. *Girls* can *be valuable!*

In their twenties, Robin secured her cousin funded housing and tried to include her socially (though it challenged the hard-won friendships she herself didn't feel secure in). Where were the parents? Well, they'd been able to retire from duties, satisfied in the knowledge that they'd made a successful appointment. 'Oh, Robin's really good at this stuff – she's better than we are at talking to professionals. Let her do it!' Robin had *learnt* to be good at talking to people in positions of authority because her own psychic survival had depended on it. So minimised was she within the family that it was only by garnering respect outside of it that she felt she had any worth at all.

WOMEN ARE <u>ANGRY</u>

When Robin's own babies were born male, she'd struggled. This had been her opportunity, she realised, to adjust a legacy, to inject a sense of value into a female baby from the get-go, to let her child feel wanted for who she actually was, in a way she'd never experienced. She came to me, not only to process her current sense of disappointment, but, more importantly, to heal from the primary, original wound of being an unwanted female.

Robin's presenting problem was physical, and she carried it physically. She'd been plagued by blinding migraines her whole life. With two babies of her own to care for, she no longer had time for the 'luxury of pain'. But Robin sensed that this was actually a psychological issue, and she wanted to treat it as such. For her, to talk was to heal. She worked her story *out*. But she also needed to do something with the physical tension in her neck and shoulders, which travelled upwards to pinch and twist the nerves around her left eye, leaving her blinded and vomiting. She'd wanted to hit out at the family who had used her, as she described it, as a 'kidney-donor' baby, as an unpaid carer. Her conditioning meant that it took her a long time – months – to come to terms with the rage she felt towards these people, who'd kept her captive to their own needs, enjoyed her sacrifices and the way that she'd sublimated herself as a mechanism of survival. We know that repressed anger may be a perpetuating factor in the pain experience. Robin seemed to know that, too. Recent scientific findings show that people with migraines or tension headaches also present with higher levels of suppressed anger and emotional distress. Robin suspected allowing the feelings to surface would ultimately help her symptom.

Once Robin had allowed herself the anger, she wanted to know, 'What can I do with this? I actually want to scream at them, punch them, ask how they could be so selfish and cruel and negligent, whilst on the surface appearing so kind and generous.' For these wounds are worn on the inside by women. These aren't the scars that child protection services or a social worker would be interested in. These days, we finally allow child carers their legitimate status. In name, at least. But the badge only tends to be applied in the most clear-cut cases. When someone is an *emotional* caregiver, when a child is silently *parentified* like this, there isn't exactly a system which swings into action to protect them. But we need to get better at acknowledging these family processes for ourselves, because they aren't uncommon. I can bring multiple examples to mind of girls being gently exploited and coerced in 'benign' ways which align with what's expected at a wider social level, and so draw no particular attention.

Robin's rage at what she had been cornered into providing her family had *become* her migraine. Neurogenic inflammation – connected to anger across many studies – is key to migraine pain production and may even begin as a response to psychological stress.

In Robin's case, she began to think of her anger as setting off the inflammation which led to her migraine episode – occurring for her at this point almost weekly.

What could she do about the pain? The inflammation felt so hot and her angrily beating heart felt as if it directly began to swell her capillaries: 'I don't even need to actively be thinking of my situation. I feel as if my mind has stored this up for a lifetime, and what I know I've been used for lies around in me. My body knows before my brain does.'

We began to talk about cold as an antidote. Robin found that laying ice blocks on her carotid artery and behind her neck, taking cold showers twice daily and visualising cold, clean rivers with her eyes closed helped to counteract the heat pulsating around her anger. Slowly, as she spoke and understood more, and stuck to her regimen of chill and icy meditation, Robin began to get on top of her rage. It stopped owning her and defining her health. She was able to axe the cycle of pain meds which was failing to do the job, and which in itself was leading to side effects. As Robin cooled down, as her breathing calmed and her shoulders relaxed, as her anger was understood and the heat of it was soothed out of her body and mind, the frequency of her migraines gradually slowed.

Cold therapies have been relied on as a treatment of migraine for over 150 years. Frozen carotid wraps around the neck have been noted in trial to significantly diminish migraine pain and were shown by recent meta-analysis to be an instantly effective migraine treatment. The landscape of anger on which Robin's migraines were built was also addressed by the use of cold, because of the physical inflammation associated with chronic levels of the emotion. As well as addressing inflammation itself through slowing of blood flow, cold therapy boosts production of both anti-inflammatory products and pro-inflammatory cytokines. If we can reduce associated inflammation, we're disrupting the feedback loop.

Robin's babyhood story, of being born into a body which would act against her, signalling to her family that it could treat her however it desired, is very familiar to my work. It's echoed, but ultimately plays through to a different outcome, with Maya.

Maya
Anger as anorexia. Her strategy = Angry art

Maya *was* the hoped-for Girl Baby. Unfortunately, her mental health bears witness to the car crash reality of this. Maya was cosseted from before birth. She talked of how her mother was afraid to walk, for fear of dislodging the embryo in her uterus. And that, when she discovered the sex of the baby she was carrying, her mother's anxiety at the prospectively delicate health of a fragile Girl Baby foetus skyrocketed.

That which her parents believed was protective, Maya found suffocating. That which they believed was caring and tender, Maya found claustrophobic and disgusting. Her mum could see no separation between herself and her frail little chick. Maya grew from a smothered infant into an eventually anorexic adolescent. All of that aggressive curtailment, that *merging*, required severance. And there was no other way but to shrink her own body away from the stifling bosom of her mother's. We know that levels of internalised anger are significantly higher in anorexic patients, as compared to control populations. Maya's case is a clear example of a Young Woman feeling constrained and disabled by her mother's intrusive focus, and needing to furiously disappear herself away.

The overidentification and feminising projections of her past *disgusted* Maya. She arrived in my clinic raging. Initially, she lashed out at me, imagining that I, too, would attempt to own her, diminish her, crush her with my ideas of what a sweet little Girl Baby was. I didn't. And this was enough for a tenuous trust to build. I held back my concerns and fought the instinct to protect, frail as this patient undeniably was. Instead, we sought to invest her with strength, to build some scaffolding inside which her rage could be housed.

Because Maya didn't have much strength to channel her impacted fury physically, she began to draw. Her sketches were not skilful, but they were raw and passionate and loaded with heavy meaning. They screamed of the trapped, stuck rage she felt, and became no less dark, but far more certain as our work went on. Her voice in therapy grew more confident, her feelings expressed with more clarity. Her body gradually grew stronger. She described how her apartment had begun to fill with her artwork and how friends had started to ask to buy pieces. She began to sell at small fairs. The point of the story isn't about material success or profit. It's about how Maya began to profit internally, and turn what had been so limiting into something which yielded riches and increased her independence and power – power which was finally directed outwards.

Our brains, for all their incredible complexity, have limited ways of presenting their suffering. Though the precise flavour of stuck emotion may be very differently experienced by each sufferer, there are relatively few pathways for that brain to express its suffering. This is why labels like 'obsessive compulsive disorder' or 'generalised anxiety disorder' actually tell us so little. And why, in treating the symptom, it's so critical to drill down into the cause.

For example, OCD would fall under the bracket for receiving treatment medically by SSRIs (antidepressants). If this doesn't help, sometimes an anti-psychotic is prescribed. This is what I mean by limitation. Just as the presenting symptom can look so narrow, we really aren't very sophisticated when it comes to medicating the most complex organ in our body. OCD diagnosed perinatally (during pregnancy or in the year following childbirth) is managed as a type of PND. Where's the person, where's the human, with all of their narrative mess, in this picture? Who, in our woefully overstretched, decimated healthcare system, has time to ask a patient about her relationship with her mother, her own babyhood, before they prescribe pills?

You see how we're approaching this in the wrong way. I'm not blaming individuals. I'm once again lamenting a *system* which thinks it's saving itself money by taking medicated shortcuts.

WOMEN ARE <u>ANGRY</u>

In which women lose out time after time. Professionals are often now too exhausted and scorched to look to evidence which could provide a better solution; a different course of treatment – for example, to wonder at the mechanisms underlying the symptom. It seems too much of a luxury to open our eyes to the elevated anger scores found in individuals presenting with symptoms of OCD. We same professionals might even respond, 'It can't be this simple! You can't blame everything on anger!' *Can't* you? It's true that 'anger' might not be the only word for this most violent and forceful of feelings. It's true that it's a catch-all, and what I really mean is aggression, violence, displeasure, dissatisfaction, hatred, frustration, irritation, full-body envy, rage, annoyance ... and every other negative emotion in between. The point is, none are available to us as women. Not really. It's neater and cleaner for people to talk in terms of 'times of the month', 'baby blues', 'bitchy' or 'perinatal OCD'. And so, this spectrum of emotion remains the one least often consciously experienced by women. Because we learn about our feelings through the language society teaches us and through the lens medicine uses, this module has most definitely been *off* the syllabus. This needs to change. Now. As an illustration of what's possible when you 'use your words', let's meet Shar and her baby, Rae.

Shar
Anger as OCD. Her strategy = Swearing

Baby Rae came in with her mum, Shar. Shar had been diagnosed with OCD and so Rae received treatment alongside her. It's a therapist's secret dream to gain access to a baby before things start to go wrong for them. As adult therapists, we normally don't get to work with babies directly. In a sense, of course we're always working with the family, but if you can get the most vulnerable of its members into the actual room – this is gold.

We had to work through Shar's rage with her own mother in order to safeguard Rae from the handed-down version, no less toxic for being wrapped up in the presenting symptom of OCD. Shar's own mother was uninvolved and chilly. She didn't see her daughter as a human person – more as a kind of embarrassment who needed to prove her worth. Poor Shar was desperate to do something different when it came to her daughter. Because our minds tend to direct us through our own early learning, and because there's no *actual* guidebook available for when your baby is born, we cast about looking for the time in our lives when the *concept of baby* registers as most familiar. For most of us, this is our own babyhood. Though we don't have conscious memories of that time, our minds do their best to kick up as much data as they have on it, and can flood us with it. Women are especially vulnerable to the impact of overwhelming unconscious events after having given birth, partly due to the fact they've been turned inside out, physically and psychologically. If their psyches try to chuck in what being a baby was like for them, they're less protected than ever. If they were scared and unheld as babies, now, as mothers, they'll probably feel the effects of that like a tsunami.

To complicate this further, we often have our own mothers still on hand, realising they screwed up back then and unconsciously (or even consciously) wanting a re-run – or maybe even floating about repeating the same mistakes. Some of us are lucky enough to have had good experiences of being a baby. But I would say only a very few – because babies are extremely demanding and what they need, as tiny helpless mammals, is to be held constantly, fed on demand and sleep tucked up next to us. Think: tiny monkey. Although I push for this, in reality, how many human mothers are able to tolerate that? When we have employers breathing down our necks and partners who only get two weeks off to help us, we probably have to accept that our babies just won't be getting what they need.

Shar's preoccupation layered on top of any basic dilemma about how she was mothering. She was so anxious to keep any hint of the rage towards her own mother out of the picture, as well as protecting Rae from the envy she felt towards her for not being baby Shar with *her* mother, that she completely squashed all treacherous and powerful feelings back inside and wore them there.

For Rae and Shar, we had to get that fury evacuated. It needed to leave that place in which it so uncomfortably-comfortably sat; in Shar's mind, but with increasing implications for Rae. Rae was beginning to have a drastically less mammalian experience of babyhood than she needed. As Shar grew increasingly caught up with repetition and what would happen if she didn't obsessively calibrate Rae's world, she became increasingly unable to give her the animal, close, messily loving experience she needed. There *is* no medication, no chemical compound for Shar's condition: a new mum with a checked-out, cauterised mother and helpless mammal-baby, who she can't care for in the straightforward way Rae needs. There's no medication. But there is treatment.

In reality, what was contaminating was not Shar's OCD. The toxic entity forcing its way into this brand-new relationship was the rage born of Shar's long-standing relationship with her own mum. And probably, if we're being realistic, this damage had been running for generations.

So, how were we to get it discharged safely now? The result was surprising. *By swearing*! When Shar learnt to call her mother a c*nt for what she'd done to her, to be able to see her cold disinterest as disastrous for a little growing mammalian Girl Baby, she began to crawl out of the intergenerational quagmire. We stumbled upon this strategy by accident. The word shot out unexpectedly in a session, when Shar was talking about how horrible someone had been to her as she was struggling to get Rae up the steps from a train platform. She then went on to directly talk about her mum, and how coldly unhelpful she'd been when Rae was born, offering nothing of warmth and only fussiness.

From there, she realised that she couldn't remember her mother ever hugging her. 'When I got my management position at the salon, she kind of *nodded* her praise? But she's never once told me she loves me. Never.' The flash of pain and dawning rage which landed was astonishing. '*She*'s the c*nt! Why would you bring another human into the world you knew you wouldn't be able to love? I know she'd say, on her deathbed, "Of course I did." But what good is that if you can't say it in life? How was I to know? Well, I didn't know. The only way I knew to get warmth was by achieving.'

Every day after this, Shar said her 'c*nts'. 'Other people do their gratitudes. Look where that got me.' Her OCD gradually began to exit stage left. The symptom was finally verbalised with something like the forcefulness with which it had been turned inwards. What was also remarkable was the improvement in her relationship with her mum. Shar was no longer frightened of her. The fearful cage placed around her was Shar's mum's best strategy in protecting her daughter from a world she felt was unsafe and punitive for women. Shar was no longer afraid to speak her mind and, freed of the locked-in rage which tunnelled itself inwards, she was also able to explore her mum's motivations for treating her this way.

GIRL BABY

So we begin to see how the way in which we treat Girl Babies, the dreams and projections we throw into them from the minute we know we're giving birth to one, shapes them forever and leaves them struggling under the weight of a set of expectations; a *brand*, which proves too much to reconcile with the messaging that later hits them. Forget all that bullshit about the world being their oyster; girls are shackled by a narrative woven into the fabric of every patriarchal institution from before they are even born. You can now see that this is where the labelling begins. The colour pink is the marker for the ideas which stack up and crowd in on the back of it.

When babies are born, we need to try to hold our 'fantasies' away whilst being absolutely tuned in and lost inside the 'reverie', which is what psychoanalysts call that locked-in gaze, where you see mums hold their baby's eyes in theirs. This obsessional regard is critical neurologically. It's where theory of mind and mental mirroring kick off – that baby understands that they are held in someone else's mind. The shared, adoring experience is helping to literally grow those parts of the brain which are capable of reaching towards and connecting with another human. This is where empathy and relating begin, which is why mums walking around glued to their phones whilst their babies desperately search around trying to make connection with some eyes is catastrophic for human development. This is why babies in orphanages hook onto light bulbs as 'mother'. Babies' brains are desperate for connection; they are starving for it. We owe our babies this. It's the basis on which their future capacity to healthily attach is founded.

If this connection is unconsciously loaded to prep girls for their later roles, with expectations that she's 'good' and 'quiet' and 'calm', we're already differentiating between her and her brother, whose demands are secretly better tolerated and indulged. In reality, she's a bunch of unformed neurons, bearing no significant differences to her brother. Repeat: there are nothing but negligible differences between boys' and girls' brains when they're born. There are more differences between the brains of *other girls*, than between boys and girls. The rest is what we do to her. The rest is the training we *don't* give her in building bricks and ball throwing. Of course, when you practise spatial tasks, you get good at them. Of course, when you only give girls pink dollies and boys construction kits, brains differentiate. Maybe the Football Association knew what it was doing with its 1921 women's football ban. Once we're unleashed, we're competition and threatening to the structures which favour men. Better for them to keep the beast contained.

What we can do for Girl Baby

As discussed, the projections begin before a baby is born. But if we know that, we can do something about it. Even if you're currently nowhere near an actual baby, you're housing the brain that belonged to the baby version of you. Thinking along these lines can help you reflect on what happened to you as a baby and whether you'd change any of your current behaviours or ideas, knowing how unhelpful they probably are to you now.

- If you're in a hetero partnership, are you asking yourselves, 'Can *we* Have It All? How can *we* do this?'

- Be prepared for society to throw curveballs by way of maternity leave and expectations about how you're going to divide your time. Part of 'doing equality' at home involves planning ahead for this.

- Bringing up babies is *so hard*. We're just trying to survive the best we can and get through the experience with everyone in one piece. But we can try to think about our pasts and what we know about how we were brought up, in order to try to be more conscious of what we're imposing.

- Scrutinise our inner sexist: who do we expect Girl Baby to be to us, and why? Stopping the intergenerational tidal wave of gendered expectation is a mammoth task ... But if the rules can be even partially rewritten on our watch, what an achievement!

- We need to try to hold our projections away from the baby and think about these feelings in ourselves instead. Is this sense of injustice at our own upbringing, which might be coming to light post-birth, something we need to resolve personally, instead of expecting another girl to shoulder?

- Watch your language. Even when she's tiny. How are you addressing Girl Baby? Is she a 'right madam' or a 'little princess' or 'an angel'? Do you find yourself referring to her crying as 'bad'? Is she only a 'good girl' when she eats and sleeps how we want her to? How do you talk to older brothers about her? Are they meant to 'look after' or 'protect' her?

- Talk about anger in an ordinary way as language develops, just as we talk about happiness and sadness, pain and excitement.
- Think about the toys you buy – mix up the spectrum. Pink is pretty, but *other colours are available*. Consider the bucketloads of gendered crap and eventual repressed rage you're handing over with it – that's not so pretty.
- Talk to infant boys about their own complex feelings. Challenge imagined expectations that you need to shield them from a more limited emotional range. If we listen carefully to them, they'll in turn become better listeners.

Right, trot off and find your little pink handbag, dolly buggy and plastic crown. We're heading for the Land of Little Girl …

CHAPTER FIVE

Little Girl

FROM GIRL BABY to Little Girl … The smooth segue of our shutdown begins to consolidate and our bodies gear up to absorbing the rage about this. Let's explore the ways in which our shutdown is paved. As a Little Girl, we're handed the tools to unconsciously perpetuate the gagging as we grow, thereby cementing our perverse relationship to rage. We apologise, we don't rock the boat. We're trained not to articulate negative feeling. We internalise our shame and guilt. Saying sorry is one of our most successful own-goals: 'Sorry for shouting, sorry for crying, sorry for ranting (talking). Sorry for existing.'

Indeed, this chapter is mainly about guilt and shame, and how society is only too willing to espouse and exploit this convenient form of internalised rage. Society stealthily nudges us into submitting to the internalised bully of our own self-blame. The pressure to be good and sweet and caring is a brilliant tool for ensuring this. We learn that 'others always come first'. Our anger is driven further inwards, where it wreaks havoc on our psychological and physiological systems. Why do we find ourselves hostage to these pressures, these sly expectations? Guilt and shame, which, in themselves, form a sort of confusing inverted fury that can't be released externally, and instead twists itself back around onto us. Whatever it is that guilt and shame both represent and mask is what we frequently have to wade through in treatment, in order to help women access the volcano of feeling underneath. Shame and guilt are a form of violation for women. Society and those around us don't actually need to do anything targeted or obvious by way of steering our behaviour. All that's required is a passive hint that we're 'too much' 'too loud' or 'too questioning'. *We* take up the inference and run with it. The case studies in this chapter show how we can teach Little Girls (including the one hidden in our adult minds, forming the foundation for all future wiring) to ditch this messaging and do it differently.

Little Girlhood is the age when we really begin to use language to express the products of our mind and give voice to the feelings our body generates in us in response to environmental events and other people's behaviours. One of the main obstacles to identifying our feelings as anger from this age is that a vocabulary isn't generally provided for it. If Girl Baby doesn't have the words, how can Little Girl then *be* angry? She must be sweet, caring, kind, thoughtful, *nice*, pretty, polite. We're not taught the language with which to express our anger, even when our older brothers use their larger size or louder voices against us. We learn how ordinary it is to be belittled and feel diminished and keep our bodies neat and within our parameters. There's simply no vocabulary for anything other than that.

Increasingly frequently, I find myself so dumbfounded at

what I'm hearing in clinic that my professional mask slips. I need to ask a woman to repeat herself. And I notice that, in repetition, she undermines her voice, quietens herself down. She assumes someone is *doubting* her feeling, rather than allowing her more space for it, and she needs little encouragement to doubt it herself: 'Maybe it's just me', 'Perhaps it wasn't that bad', 'They were probably right.' The basic position women take up is one which screams 'I'm wrong!' Her thought is the wrong one, her feeling is unreliable, her instinct can't be trusted, her behaviour is doubtless going to get her into trouble. And it seems that an unbroken thread connects this sensation to childhood.

There's a stricture on self-expression and pushing her ideas to the fore, for fear of looking not just silly, but deeply *wrong*; that she hasn't grasped something, or has the wrong end of the stick. These feelings of wrongness run deep. They quickly turn to shame and, before we know it, women have erased themselves apparently voluntarily from the social arena. Little Girl is when the seeds are planted for a woman avoiding a particular job application because she won't be good enough or isn't qualified – or because, if she does get it, she'll mess it up in some way and it's all too exposing. Great! There's a man waiting who can do it. It all works perfectly. And it starts from this point. Not to sound completely joyless (OK, a bit joyless), a recent study involving gender messaging in children's stories proved thought-provoking on the topic of continued teaching of passivity in Little Girls. It reminds us of how many expected gender behaviours are subtly present in our go-to favourites, and of how suggestible young children are to the messaging that we, as adults, can choose to screen out. The following case study demonstrates just how influenced we are by covert signalling.

Juno
Anger as damaging relationships. Her solution = Writing

Juno is a great example of a patient who *appeared* to have received the messaging that girls *can* speak up, that they *can* claim their space. Her unconventional experience of a childhood spent outside of the usual nuclear strictures could have enabled her entrance into a more equal adult experience. But it didn't.

Juno was a journal-writer. I always encourage my patients to journal. It sounds so naff and trite, and I loathe the beige-ness of the word – which is why I prefer to label it 'observation'. Let's throw science at it. Forcing yourself to free-associate for ten minutes a day is actually a great way of both introspecting and processing. 'Stream of consciousness' writing was a concept coined in 1892 by the psychologist William James as a way of accessing the dynamic and covert products of the mind. Some of my patients do this between sessions and call their notebooks names like 'my pocket therapist' or 'my brain on the outside'. Some of them bring their diaries with them. Some of them draw, some write poems. Some show me things they've read that week or found online which seem to articulate their experience – especially at the beginning of therapy, when finding words to capture the extent of the emotion can be difficult. Whatever helps women express their feelings, however they feel they can best communicate it, counts; it's all grist for the mill.

Juno needed to write. It helped her to separate things

out – an activity I urge patients to strive for. I do it myself. Writing is like breathing for me. If I can't write, my brain suffocates and atrophies. The technique begins with the separation of thoughts from feelings, which sounds basic, but we're really not taught how to do this, typically, from childhood. And it often scuppers us for our whole lives. When we've got better at doing this, we can then move on to the importance of separating issues from one another and working out how we want to manage them.

Juno's life had always been somewhat chaotic, growing up in an artily bohemian family with few apparent constraints. Juno had discovered sex and drugs at a very young age, and her lack of internal boundaries was reflected in the dysregulated relationships she began to form. The fluid home life she was raised in was, in fact, an institution to 'benevolent sexism'. Her mother appeared to be cherished and deified. The ability to bear children was seen as an almost saintly act. Women's beauty and earthy 'intuition' were worshipped. Again, this is all very flattering, but quite disabling in practice. Juno's dad became more and more successful professionally, but, via his fawning and adulation, Juno's mother was consciously or unconsciously coerced into the role of domesticity over artistic output.

Although her mum was a feminist on paper and inducted Juno into concepts of equality, there wasn't much modelling of how this might play out in the real world. It certainly wasn't in evidence at home, where her mum had six children to contend with. Here, even though her dad seemed to defer to her mum in all matters, what Juno witnessed was a woman chained to the sink in a really conventional way; more, in fact, than many of Juno's friends' mums, who were out working in offices. Her dad also had a way of completely erasing his Little Girl. He didn't look at the artwork she made; he didn't come to parents' evenings and hear how well she was doing. Her efforts to impress him and persuade him to respect what he saw were pointless. Whilst he talked the talk of cherishing and hearing and praising her talents, his behaviour was inhibiting. His envy of the next generation's potential, and sense that his position as the Special One might be under threat, meant he could only withhold.

As she looked back, Juno saw that this muddle had really instructed her in the veneration of men's creativity and power. You see the problem. Something which looked so progressive was quietly reinforcing the opposite.

Another issue for Juno as a Little Girl was the taboo on anger. In this quiet, intellectual household, the rawness of rage had no place. Juno barely even knew that feeling had a name. She'd definitely felt it; something bubbling up inside at how she was 'deeply respected' and eulogised. It all felt so *ick*. But Juno had no expression for it. She started to cut her body to try to force exit some of what she housed inside. She could even look back at her journal later and realise that she'd been trying to express something which completely eluded her. On paper, Juno's home circumstances might sound unusual to most of us, but they highlight in clearer terms something I'm sure many of us relate to: the sensation of being a furious and confused Little Girl, with no words for your emotion and no one and no place to house it.

When Juno moved to London to study at art college, she began to discover the true impact of her allegedly sexism-free girlhood. Growing up in an environment which boasted emancipation, which saw itself as above the conventions and bounds of gender, but which was actually near-biblical in its traditional role allocation, had robbed her of the tools to identify poor treatment now. She was just completely ill-equipped. Writing had helped her to make sense of her decisions and behaviours. But when she came to me, she was completely confused: 'I'm a feminist! I expect men to treat me as an equal!' But here she was, bruised from another man who'd envied her and sliced her up psychologically, in order to feel some power. The therapeutic tool of her writing 'just wasn't cutting it anymore'. She was ready to confront her feelings and needed to work through the clash of Little Girl early-years messaging with her actual, lived adult reality.

What began to emerge in the therapy was dichotomous. Although her own feminist values were, in part, built on the freedom she saw her mother exercise, Juno understood that she also felt very angry about the lack of structure, boundaries and predictability that she'd experienced growing up. She appreciated that much of her own creativity and free-spiritedness emanated from her upbringing, but that she had also often felt neglected, lost and unseen. Here was a feminism with no substantial core – more lip service, in a sense.

The type of relationships she'd chosen for herself seemed to follow a pattern of creative men who placed their own needs and ambitions before her. Feeling unimportant and insignificant was a state of being for Juno, which she accepted as normal. Her anger came through as the self-harm she subjected herself to and through investment in these diminishing relationships. Juno began writing back to herself as a child. Through tapping into decades-old feelings of outrage and confusion, Juno began to feel her own self-worth. She began to see how her feelings had been justified. From her adult perspective, she could now see that the modelling she'd received about what it was to be a woman was weird and contradictory.

Watching Juno blossom as she permitted herself her own feelings of anger was often frustratingly non-linear, but ultimately gratifying. Over time, Juno gradually saw the positive effects of her growing confidence shape her professional output. When she eventually established a long-term partnership, with a man to whom she felt equal, we both understood that something lasting had been achieved. The Little Girl who'd been taught that women were creative deserts had finally understood the truth – and had used her historic indignation as fuel for productivity.

Who here, like Juno, has ever felt shut down, talked across, condescended or outright ignored? What do you feel about that? Possibly, you're numb to it. You're inured. Because it's something which becomes familiar from Little Girlhood. Our real needs begin to go unheard, our volume gets dialled down for the first time, we're squashed and our ideas are diminished ... We get used to surrendering space. Perhaps you've spent an evening, a career or a lifetime being *mansplained* to. This happens in subtle ways within marriage or families, too. In Little Girlhood, it's found that families praise male siblings in a different way, which contributes to confidence behaviours later. My patients frequently admit that, as Little Girls, their parents had higher expectations of them in areas like tidiness and kindness, simply because they were female. It's all just so boring – that the biases of these youngest years can still hold such sway in adulthood, as we bow and scrape, apologising for our existence; feeling as if our role is to sort and smooth.

In enduringly familiar scenarios, mothers and daughters take up the role of unwilling stooge, the recipient of eye-rolling and gently denigrating comments ('must be the time of the month', 'Mummy can't do numbers/maps', 'you're *nagging* again'). Such comments become concretised within the ecosystem of a household. I'm astonished to hear women – strong-seeming women with invincibly shiny careers – talk today of how the gendered roles persist across management of finances and domestic duties. In these moments, I can only conclude we really haven't moved on much since the fifties. Since these messages are internalised by Little Boy as well as Little Girl, we're presumably looking at at least another generation's assumption that this is the way things shake down.

WOMEN ARE <u>ANGRY</u>

As our *passive* Little Girl grows, it makes sense that she might linger too long in more junior roles (in an infantilised, apologetic position) and isn't as far ahead as she could be when she takes maternity leave (during which, male counterparts are receiving promotions). She loses time, she's on the back foot, even if she returns to work more determined and possibly capable from her experience of mothering. The point is, we know all this statistically, but I'm hearing the individual accounts daily of *why* women are minimising themselves. Of where it began in childhood, in being made to feel silly or attention-seeking or labelled as show-offs or 'little madams' if their voices were raised too loudly. And it makes for bleak listening. A great article by Alena Papayanis in *HuffPost* says it all. Being nice, kind and socialised into people-pleasing ultimately led to a complete alienation of her needs. Devastatingly relatable.

As the years go by, I'd have expected to hear these narratives diminish, that my generation would have cracked it: smashing through glass ceilings, narrowing the gap, gaining in confidence and watching the successes stack up; joyously benefitting from the alleged structures and policies designed to ensure our success. Instead, it feels as if I'm watching women get to a certain point before they're chewed up and spat out by a system which has had enough of kowtowing to feminism and equality, but which is now slick at talking the talk.

And, if Little Girl sees her mum struggling with these same dynamics, however subtle, she unconsciously identifies with them and ultimately complies on some level. Though this doesn't stop the rage from building. Patients of my age have spoken to me about how incredulous they used to feel at these role allocations as they grew up. At school, we were told: you can be astronauts! And vets! And surgeons! Which was strange, in a way, because we didn't know any women who *were* those things. Clearly, there wasn't really a language for voicing our misgivings. We had to hold the two realities in tandem and accept them. It was just *normal*. The Little Girl versions of the adults in my practice had watched their mums washing and cooking and shopping and taking care of younger siblings, just the same as in all previous generations. Though their mum *may* have had a paid job too, normally home was where most of her hours were spent. It doesn't matter about the messaging at school, kids learn through observation, from which we deduce patterns about how the world works.

One patient remembers, when she'd been a Little Girl, trying to talk to her mum about 'Why Daddy doesn't cook dinner.' But her mum replied, 'Well, Dad just gets home later than me – it makes sense that we do it this way.' Her mother was a teacher, not because she was particularly passionate about teaching, but because, having completed university, she knew she needed to get a job which enabled her to take care of a family. This woman had looked around in the seventies, seen how few options there were for retaining any kind of financial stake and made a 'sensible choice' which took no account of her own desires and left her stuck in a repeating pattern of trying to juggle work and home life. Which, judging by my patients' stories, has set a robust precedent for subsequent generations.

Though, on a macro level, we can point to women rocking leadership roles in male-dominated industries, and so on, what

I hear in practice is the granular reality of how stuck these habits still are, and how detrimental they are to our health. Nowadays, 41 per cent of UK women work full-time (as opposed to 25 per cent in 2010). In the US, it's 37.3 per cent. But with not much less to do on the domestic front. According to a 2022 article in the *Guardian*, women in heterosexual couples are still completing 65 per cent of the household chores. A CBS report suggests that even so-called 'breadwinner' wives spend around three and a half hours more a week than husbands on house-work and care provision.

As well as what we're modelled, something else is going on in our gendered attitude to kids, which lines them up for this legacy. 'Boys will be boys' is the apparently unshakeable view which sets us up to look at each other differently. There's still a perception that Little Girl, as she grows, is more dependable, sensible and useful than her brother, or boys in her class, which children themselves buy into. This differentiation is dressed up as some sort of compliment: 'You're so much more *emotionally intelligent/empathic/instinctive!*' But, actually, this seems to be another stealth message which shackles women to a life of care and responsibility. It doesn't matter how many years we spend educating ourselves or earning – our primary function in families is as feeder and carer, and this still seems to be the role which garners most focus in our lives. What I notice amongst female patients is just how often we seem to sleepwalk into this set-up, and how early the obligations begin. How can we have travelled so far from our mothers' reality of scant professional choice – we've done it! We *are* the surgeons and the astronauts (well, a few of us are, trying to screen out the sexual harassment as we go) – and yet have wound up in this place of broken burnout?

Little Girls are taught to nurture and be gentle. Caretaking is written into our education. Many in my patients' lives still appear to doubt that women can be logical, that they can think rationally and entrepreneurially. From birth, we're seen as emotionally adept and sensitive. Our brothers, generally, are not. We're also deemed to be self-contained and psychologically capable. Baffling that, on the one hand, we're painted as frail and ill-equipped, yet, when it suits everyone else, we're leant on as dependable and stoic. Since the expectation is that we're so self-contained and undemanding, we must find our own ways of regulating our pain. It's ironic that men are seen to be the emotionally repressed ones when we've been pushing down this rage since we got left in the caves to dust the mammoth skins. *Fact.*

As a *modern-day* example of the hardwired caring expectation, one patient was angered by her father's insistence that she take a holiday from work and come to stay with them 'for a rest'. She well knew what this would involve, since her mother was severely disabled (she'd already had an active involvement in getting these parents the support they needed medically, though, of course, they'd turned away the actual carer she'd found them). Another patient told of how, after suffering a minor accident, her mother had said, 'You can't let anything happen to you! We need you!' This patient had young children who would undoubtedly be the worst affected by injury occurring to their mother. That's not how her parents saw it, though. You see how the system just keeps on keeping on? Neither of these women pointed out the flaws in the statements, as they knew it would 'upset people' and start an argument. And they'd been trained, as Good Little Girls, that this wasn't an option.

This is a nice time to return to the idea of how impacted, chronic anger appears to lend itself to states of internal inflammation, and what the effect of this looks like, as far as our mental health is concerned.

My experience of working with Nadia is a good illustration.

Nadia
Anger as depression. Her strategy = Violence

Nadia blocked it all. At the beginning of our work together, she blocked my every attempt to make contact. The one element in her life she was proud of was her career. She worked in account management , and she was respected. To a degree. She'd recently discovered that her salary was significantly less than men in her team (some of whom were younger and not as experienced as her). Her rage about this was the reason she'd sought therapy. 'I trust you'll be able to help me fix this,' was her aggressive challenge. She had no trust at all. And I felt her disdain keenly. Nadia was brusque, intimidating and entirely miserable. She'd been married briefly in her early thirties, but 'didn't see the point' of staying in such an 'ineffectual' relationship. I could see that, if I didn't pass muster, I, too, would be relegated to the realms of the ineffectual.

Nadia was prickly and rejecting and strangely

compelling. She kept me on my toes always and was brutally challenging towards anything I offered. In essence, she made me *sweat*. She loved to torture me – as, I quickly realised, life had felt tortuous to her. She'd been desperately unpopular at school and her parents had treated her in a both cosseting and negligent way, preoccupied with her physical well-being and neglecting her psychological health. She herself drew the conclusion that this was connected to her gambling-addicted older brother. There was a 12-year age gap between them and she knew that he'd been the apple of her mum's eye. A 'spoilt brat', she'd concluded. Even as a Little Girl, she remembered being horrified at the way he spoke to her parents, and could feel the disdain he held them in. She felt a sense of responsibility to give them a different experience her time around. But also a resentment that she needed to. She brought this resentment into my consulting room *wholesale*.

As we crawled along through the treacle of the work, one step forward, three back, we realised the extent to which the suffocation of her parents' anguish had impacted Nadia. And Nadia was offended and crushed by this. She was both never enough, and too much. The innocence of her mind and her good behaviour were a source of potential terror for her parents, but they also invoked a certain kind of envy. They needed to protect her from whatever had seized their son, but they also resented the way her solid existence shone a light on his instability. She was always being asked to 'understand' and 'forgive' him, somehow implying to her that 'it was all right for her' – she didn't suffer in life as he did. Whereas, as Nadia saw it, it was only taking the difficult path of discipline and conscientiousness which had differentiated them as siblings. Finally, Nadia grew sick of it. She herself felt fury at her brother, whose destructive behaviours cast a shadow. After a life spent trying to please and feeling rage that she should have to, with no recognition for how hard she'd worked – both in her life and for her parents – she arrived in my consulting room angrily suicidal. Something of the rage at her brother's unapologetic, purposeful feeling of destructiveness had gotten into her own behaviour. As if she wanted to finally give someone else a taste of how she'd been made to feel – both under intolerable pressure and not good enough. Therapy was her chance.

Nadia was brutalised by the trap she'd felt caught in from girlhood. Her cold fury at the injustice of her brother's legacy was tangible. She wore it like a coat. She wrapped herself up in it by day and slept with it like a blanket at night. But she was dutiful. She was a Good Little Girl, so wouldn't rebel and leave these parents to suffer alone. She bore it so they didn't have to. But, of course, emotions don't work like that. Her parents still felt it. Their pain, exasperation and confusion were like a fountain which replenished itself constantly. And Nadia felt her role was forever to mop up the eternally refilling well. As her brother's life wound itself around ever more chaotic and risky experiences, Nadia felt increasing pressure to root herself to her parents and their emotional needs. But her anger and resentment about this had to go somewhere.

My work with Nadia was slow and painful. Many times, she hated me for representing someone who apparently came between herself and the opportunity of death. It caused *me* pain to be so reviled and denigrated. But this wasn't really my pain, it was hers. It was the pain of years, the rage of a lifetime.

I encouraged Nadia to start throwing things: ice cubes onto the patio, wet washcloths in the shower, stones onto a pebble path. At first, she felt self-conscious and flung her shame back onto me: 'What a stupid idea! You're encouraging violence! Aren't you meant to be helping me find peace, or some bollocks?' But eventually, in tandem with the gentle but persistent therapeutic work of uncovering the damage done in her youth, Nadia felt the benefits.

After a few months of working together, I wondered whether she might formalise her explosive physical expressions. Together, we decided she'd try kick-boxing. As she gained in confidence and began to form friendships with those in her class, she decided to go further, and joined an extreme sports programme. She started going on fitness retreats, which sounded brutal but seemed to align with the extremity of her internal experience. Eventually, she met a man on one of the camps, with whom she began a relationship. Without the therapy and our watchful united eye, I'm certain Nadia would have killed this off too.

WOMEN ARE <u>ANGRY</u>

Nadia's depression was a deep, inverted rage. By finding release through activity, she was able to physicalise some of the energy and create enough space for more objective self-appraisal. It also enabled room for the therapeutic relationship to embed. Something about the deepening of our relationship, of the trust in me, meant that she began to slowly pull away from the iron grip of her parents' claustrophobic and accusatory panic. As the separation grew, she was, in turn, less affected by the projections.

After three years of working together, Nadia came off her antidepressant medication, which she'd been taking in ever-increasing amounts for 30 years. Three years on and her friendship circle has widened. She now sees her parents every few months, and lightly keeps in touch throughout the week. She's still in a relationship with Mark, the man she met at the camp, and hopes one day to be able to 'take the risk' of moving in with him. She talks openly now about anger, whether the deeply experienced, calcified kind which she came to call 'Neville' or the everyday irritations experienced at work by people she still has a tendency to label 'morons'. She sees her depression as being entirely comprised of rage, and feels that, in finally externalising her lifelong anger, she's been able to release herself from its inverted form. Nadia left the job which she realised didn't value her and set up professionally on her own. Though this wasn't the employment battle she'd envisaged she needed my help with, she decided her angry energy was better directed at getting her own dreams realised.

Nadia had been caught in a Little Girl state of locked-in

rage. As an adult, this presented as something more stuck and depressive. She hadn't been shown a way of expressing those feelings at the time and so had no tools to do it as an adult. As we saw in the first part of the book, depression and anger share a comparable chemical substrate, bound by inflammation and forever to be confused.

I believe that anxiety is similarly misunderstood. Psychologists have long felt that the shared physiological characteristics of anxiety and anger indicate an overlapping psychic space. As was demonstrated by the 'emotion interpretation' experiments of the sixties, our bodies have limited ways of expressing complex feeling states. Raised heart rate, tense muscles, tightness of chest and tension headaches are commonly associated symptoms of both anger and anxiety. Both moods are powered by washes of adrenaline and cortisol. Either one might be connected to a sense of lost control or lack of security so that, when confronted with a stimulus lying outside your sphere of knowledge, there may well be some trepidation, some sense of raised threat. As this sensation becomes further suffused with hormones, a feeling of being affronted, offended or angered may arise. This part will likely get ignored in women, in favour of aligning with the initial flood of intimidated overwhelm. For example, a manager at work yells at you. Hijacked by the physical freeze of this, you have little chance to explore the audacity of such treatment in a so-called professional setting. Countless times over now, I find myself helping women work through their instinctively fearful feelings, to ultimately get in touch with something much more akin to fury or outrage. We were simply not taught to do this when we were Little Girls, but it's never too late to learn. As was the case with Candy.

Candy
Anger as shyness. Her strategy = Conversation

Candy provided another really special opportunity to help gently intervene with a Little Girl, and where her path seemed to be headed to deleterious result. Candy had a three-year-old daughter, Skye. Skye was exhibiting some aggressive outbursts towards her mum, which scared Candy and caused her to revert to language which really didn't seem to be helping and which felt entirely sculpted within the socialised conventions of 'Be nice!', 'Be a Good Little Girl', 'You need to calm down.' For Skye, 'naughty step' became the answer to everything, from playing roughly with her dolls to 'answering back' or throwing toys.

Interestingly, Candy had come to therapy to work on her low self-esteem and shyness. She felt it was holding her back at a career level, and was also probably contributing to the marriage in which she felt taken for granted. As we tackled these feelings, Candy began to notice that she was projecting onto her own daughter the same disempowering habits which had been forced onto her. She remembered that, when she was little herself, she'd actually been 'quite loud' and that her parents had meanly called her the 'demanding baby'.

LITTLE GIRL

Apparently, Candy's little sister had been a 'very Good Little Girl' and she'd not really heard the end of it. You know how, in families, legends get established of how you were when you were little? And it's as if this is how most family members continue to relate to you, even when you're a grown adult? As a therapist, I *deplore* this way of completely entrapping someone within the confines of their childhood. In our first five years of life, billions of neuronal connections are forming. Little Girlhood offers families a window of opportunity to shape the healthiest trajectory for our development and build us an optimal foundation. It's helpful if a family can hold in mind that they're building the foundation for future generations, because, one day, this Little Girl might also mother her own Little Girl. She won't be a cutey little dot forever. Remembering that can help us get unstuck from the 'they're a naughty little thing' approach. This person, who's tiny now, will be taking this same brain through to adulthood. Remember the earlier point, about how the closest thing our brains have to a guidebook is information from our own past? If families could make this 'teaching' constructive and useful to us, they can really set us up to parent well ourselves (if we still want to parent, after all this! Sorry if I'm making it look unappealing – it's a hazard of the job).

Infants, as we know, are not 'good' or 'bad'. Their behaviour is not malicious. It's all survival-based. So, if a baby needs to scream to get heard, there's a reason for it. If their body tells them they need food or warmth, they believe they will die if they don't get it now. They need to be programmed that way, since they're entirely vulnerable and dependent. And some babies are just 'higher need' babies with parents who don't have the capacity to accommodate this.

Sadly, Candy was educated to believe she was *too much*, and her rage and hurt about this became impacted and internalised into an aggressive shyness which made others feel uncomfortable. I felt this in the room with her. There were a lot of silences, and it was all pretty painful, I'll confess. Like an attack. But, slowly, she began to find her voice. We forged ordinary conversations around feelings, in which we started to explore the sense of indignation about her own childhood, the slightly villainous role she'd been cast in and the way in which shame about this had robbed her of her voice.

I really need to reiterate at this point how plastic (capable of structural reorganisation) our brains are. By which I mean they're able to rewire in ways that seem utterly remarkable. Recruiting different, surprising pathways which people wouldn't have felt themselves capable of subtly, over time, can yield such fundamental change that a person feels their responses are completely different. The idea isn't to go for a personality transplant, more of a *feelings* expansion. I really want to inspire you as a reader to understand how possible this is. Though we're *compelled to repeat*, when we understand where these unhealthy drivers come from, we can liberate ourselves and think about fostering a different set of responses.

This chapter has thematically mostly dealt with women

feeling guilty about things that weren't their fault, apologising for her superior creativity over a man and allowing him therefore to overshadow her (as with Juno). Or trying to make other people feel bad to shift some of it (in the case of Nadia), or telling themselves they're doing a terrible job (Candy). Put together, I think the reason women feel so readily guilty is to do with how convinced we are that we're taking up too much space. Our defence is to be decorative, to wear beautiful clothes we're not allowed to get dirty; and if we try to get our voices heard, we are readily accused of 'bossiness'. Playground space is dominated by football games whilst we're forced into corners we can only use for talking. It's no wonder that our 'emotional faculties' become so overdeveloped, whilst expectations on boys' same 'soft skills' are so meagre. These limiting narratives are so pervasive that our brains begin to adapt around them. Taking up any room, asking for anything, trying to get our actual needs met … it all starts to feel audacious and rude. And we're made to feel bad for it. What we think of as our 'guilt' feels more like being conditioned to minimise the centimetres of planet we occupy. This persistent template of imposed diminishment needs to be instilled somehow. Higher emotional standards are drummed into us. You will empathise and take responsibility for others' feelings! At all times! If you do that, we'll let you stand on this bit of Earth. Yikes. Poor Little Girl!

These fabulous female patients – Juno, Nadia and Candy – all eventually reconfigured their assumptions. I'm not saying this process churns out perfect humans (who wants those, anyway?), but I am saying – wow, they felt better for it. *And so could you.*

What we can do for Little Girl

These aren't only steps for helping *actual* Little Girls. We all have that same Little Girl inside of us, who probably needs to hear this. And, if you're actively parenting a real-life Little Girl right now, remember that the act of caretaking can be reparative. We often parent ourselves when we parent.

- Remember that children are built to constantly observe their environment. We need to walk the walk. Look at the messages we're reinforcing if 'Daddy always drives' or 'Mummy always holds the sick bowl'. Kids create rules around repeated behaviours.
- Stop putting kids in pigeonholes within families.
- As with babies, we need to stop calling children 'good' for being quiet.
- Parents are more lenient when boys are physically aggressive. Think about this.
- Talk to girls about their anger. Let them express it. Help them find words for it. There are hundreds.
- Talk to boys about *their* anger, and expect them to be able to just as well flex their vocabulary around it.
- Be compassionate with ourselves if we think we're reinforcing something from our pasts which we really didn't intend to. This shit is hard. Saying sorry as a parent is powerful and much more constructive than wallowing in guilt.
- Make sure that we gently expect the same behaviours

of boys as girls. If there are any developmental differences, we don't need to exaggerate them, and they won't be blanket anyway – each individual develops differently within typical trajectories.

- Also, remember that both girls *and* boys like playing dollies. Only boys call them 'action figures'. Barbie can rescue people and skydive too.

- Talk about feelings – especially the uncomfortable ones – *all the time*.

- Teach little boys to listen. If we've prioritised their feelings, they'll have an internal working model for prioritising those of others.

- Talk about mums and dads and roles and how we need to try to balance these, but how sometimes the wider world makes it hard to do so.

Right, where are your too-tiny shorts and inappropriate crop tops? You're going to need them, as we veer straight into the glitter-strewn years of Queen Tween …

CHAPTER SIX

Tween Girl

IN THIS CHAPTER, we unpick the way girls and women begin to relate to each other. And how, from this age, through cute crushes on pop stars and YouTubers, we're apparently forced into certain ways of relating to men. In truth, these behaviours of tribalism and in-group hostility actually *attempt* to serve important functions. By exploring what mechanisms like bitching provide us with, we come to see why these modes of communication *appear* to give us a channel for expressing aggressive thoughts. The issue is that we're not usually directing these feelings towards the people who need to hear them. In general, we're either absolutely terrible at confrontation or a 'total bitch'. This is because we've never been granted permission by society, nor a vocabulary, to easily express our angry feelings.

In our Tween Girl years, betwixt the simplicity of Little Girlhood and the turbulence of adolescence, our raw emotions begin to translate themselves into more differentiated feelings of competition, possessiveness, sadism, resentment, envy and contempt. Even hatred. These more sophisticated feelings, which look so far from anger, appear to protect us from the socially destructive expression of pure rage, at a life stage where socially conforming begins to reign supreme. But the force of that feeling is still there, informing the intensity of these other secondary habits. Anyone with a Tween Girl in their vicinity knows that this is the age where it all kicks off.

This is when boys and girls are first divided socially. For Tween Girl, her aggression needs to move rapidly underground. More covert tactics of belonging and survival are favoured, which is where society can ramp the Little Girl guilt up a notch. Self-blame and self-recrimination are familiar states to me, as a therapist to so many women attempting to navigate the impossibilities of 'living her best life'. Yet, as we've seen, guilt in itself is a type of inverted rage, another way of 'cleaning up' after oneself – of not making a mess with one's feelings, but tucking the edges in neatly so nothing spills out.

We're so brilliant at handling uncomfortable feelings that we absorb them, even if they aren't actually our responsibility. It's as if we are rendered from some tough generation of reinforced composite. 'I'm so stupid, I'm an idiot' … we tell ourselves. Well, *some*one is, but that person may not be able to handle the truth. And isn't everyone else's happiness the priority? Because if *they*'re happy, *you*'re safe.

How many of us have, since Tweenhood, when we might have been old enough to be conscious of it for the first time, witnessed the frailty of men, of their anxieties, their terrors, and seen how, if they're not placated, these fears externalise themselves aggressively in the form of shouting, swearing or lashing out – sometimes physically; certainly, using the mass of their larger form to intimidating effect? We learn to pour water on the fire; we learn to take the hit. We see our grandmothers, mothers, aunts, older sisters and friends do it, and so we do it ourselves. We diminish and sublimate our own feelings and experiences, until we convince ourselves that we shouldn't take up the minimal space we occupy.

You can see where the idea of shrinking our bodies through controlling our size starts to come in, can't you? And you can also see where the anger would start to build in response to our necessarily suppressed reactions. This sense of not being entitled to our feelings is what contributes to suppression and symptom formation. If we slip up, if we start to feel we haven't done a good enough job in allowing others their reality, our self-blame contributes to this inverted rage. It becomes imperative that the truth of others is prioritised, since this is the safest way of ensuring our own survival. The trouble is, we may be inflicting irreparable harm to ourselves in the process.

Tweenhood marks the point at which we're really aware of what's expected of us, of how those spatial parameters will be defined. The adult version of this involves women patients explaining their position, whether she's describing her political viewpoint, a situation with families or friends, or the life choices she's made. She apologises for running overtime in a session, for 'ranting' (talking), for making me feel sad about something she's described to me. I'm continually struck by the amount of apologising women do in the consulting room, as compared with men.

There's a sense around a man's emerging therapeutic narrative that he's surprised by his emotions. *But he doesn't then (normally) apologise for them.* Women, experiencing similar feelings (issues with relationships, friendships, colleagues or family) will almost always say sorry for the perceived smallness of their troubles – reflective of how she is out there, in the wider world. One woman described how she'd said, 'No, sorry' to protestors outside an abortion clinic who'd tried to give her a leaflet. She felt enraged – but *with herself* – for not having told them what she thought of them.

From Tween Girl onwards, she learns to fit the mould. Follow that popstar, buy this sequinned training bra, *align*, stay in the huddle. Don't push outwards, where people might have to make space for you. Which is *embarrassing*. As an adult in her therapy, she feels easily self-indulgent, that someone else must be more deserving of her session; that she's wasting my time and I must see people with far worse problems. 'Sorry for coming to therapy. Sorry for forcing you to listen. Sorry for existing ...' To this, I give you Kanya.

Kanya
Anger as anxiety. Her strategy = Feminism

Kanya is a great example of someone who learnt to expand her Tween parameters, and converted her packed-down anger into something beneficial for her future. Kanya began attending therapy with me for help with her crippling anxiety. She was working in events at the time. The area in which she worked was very male, and she'd begun her employment there aged 18. The experiences she'd suffered at the hands (literally) of these men were extreme and deeply shocking. Her vulnerability had been determined in Tweenhood.

Kanya had been recruited into a caring role by her family from the outset, as the eldest of five children. Her tendency to put others first and please was her chief vulnerability, and really kicked off in her Tween years, when her family began to see her as old enough to take responsibility. Since her wired-in duty was to serve, how was she to stand up to the harassment of the men she worked with? It seemed she couldn't win. If she humoured the offender, the entire staff seemed to take this as affirmation she was in a relationship with him. If she didn't, she was terrified for her safety (possibly correctly, based on the reported behaviours of her male co-workers on feeling humiliated or rejected).

The rage Kanya was aware she felt fought with the terror and became a toxic combination internally. She began to experience acute stomach pains alongside her anxiety, for which the GP ruled out a physiological basis, and encouraged her instead to come forward for therapy. The first thing the therapy allowed Kanya was a space to express the feelings she couldn't really take anywhere else. The fact of having gone to a religious girls' school meant Kanya had never had to face the reality of being disempowered by men outside of her home environment. But being treated as nothing more than a servant in her household meant Kanya had no confidence with which to tackle the forced sexual contact at work.

Once she'd begun to vocally express the overpowering

and heavy feelings which had become the hallmark of so much of her life, Kanya started to feel physically better. But she was on the hunt for answers. A lot of her rage stemmed from the feeling she'd been thrown into a lion's den, in terms of the socially condoned behaviours of the men at her workplace. None of these men were reprimanding the others; none were seeking to ensure her protection – just as her family at home had deprioritised her well-being over their own requirements of her.

Through therapy, she began to knit together a different sense of her rights and needs. And then a friend who was at university lent her a book: Chimamanda Ngozi Adichie's *We Should All Be Feminists*. Kanya seemed to find a bedrock for a possible self-identity which could encompass her religious beliefs, but also teach her how to formulate arguments internally around how her younger years had left her so exposed to later violating behaviours. This understanding, coupled with the bolstering Kanya received through being psychologically contained in the therapy, helped knit together a sense of possibility and self-ownership. She joined a Young Feminists group in London, with many members who felt in their own ways disillusioned and silenced, and needed to find a place to talk safely. Eventually, Kanya decided to take up a degree through the Open University. Since childhood, her mind had only been celebrated in terms of its capacity to enable the desires of others. Now, it could begin to operate as a tool to protect and steer her own desires. And what about the job? She left it, and is actually leaning on the advice of the group to help her file harassment charges. The problematic point here is that Kanya had to change *her* behaviour in order to challenge the hatred she encountered. Women – yet again – doing the work. As I help trawl through, trying to support women find their voice and understand that they're not wrong, I'm endlessly struck by this irony. 'Boys will be boys ...'

Zara's Tween story began at the other extreme.

Zara
Anger as shame. Her strategy = To confront the perpetrator

Zara had grown up in a cosy family in the Midlands suburbs, with parents and a school that seemed to support her and see her, and want to help her become a Young Woman able to capably make her way in the world. Zara didn't anticipate that this expectation of unconditional championing could be exploitable later on. Her own uncomplicated Tweenhood, attending a celebrated co-ed grammar school which emphasised girl power, equipped her with a sense that nothing was beyond her reach.

Once she began as a junior in a big London marketing firm, she began to find out that the promises of girl power were pretty flimsy. A senior partner at the firm began to groom her and ask her to go to late-night dinners so he could advise on her career. At the point I met Zara, she was spinning out and confused. This man was charismatic, married and violent. He liked to tie up Zara during sex. Zara wasn't sexually experienced, but from what she'd seen online thought this must be playful. I met her at the point she was becoming scared. She'd quelled all of her terror previously, because the fear of losing her career at this point, with all her parents' pride at stake, was greater. The Good Little Girl conditioning underlying the Tween Girl, faux-emancipatory nineties messaging was exposed: 'Rude not to.' 'Mustn't be vanilla.' Where was Girl Power now?

The week before we met, Zara had tried to call an end to the relationship. In response, her boss had punched a wall. Zara was feeling disgusted with herself, frightened and stuck. She was afraid of losing her job and she was afraid of what he might do to her if she tried to break it off again. As we spoke through what had happened to her, she began to admit that she was deeply ashamed.

'Ashamed?' I asked. 'You were the victim of a serious abuse of power.'

She panicked: 'But I'm an adult! I did wrong, too!'

I explained that affairs aren't illegal, but that coercing a junior colleague into sex would certainly not be viewed favourably. He had more to lose, which was why he was using tactics of threat. Zara admitted that she still couldn't find the words to adequately convey the sense of injustice she felt, that it was easier to internalise the feelings, which is where they seemed to take the form of shame.

We tried to find the words together. And they were raw; cries of confusion from some part of her she'd never needed to know – from an overwhelmed Tween Zara, who'd been told that girl power would spell woman power. Slowly, Zara began to understand that not all adults are trustworthy. That they won't all respect her in the way she'd been taught to expect. And that she could feel very, very angry about this. Zara decided not to mention the relationship to HR (or even, frankly, report his behaviours to the police), but instead chose to have a meeting with the perpetrator in a glass room in the middle of the office. She enjoyed the way he squirmed as she read out the piece she'd prepared in therapy. Zara found a way back, at least partially, to honour that Tween version of herself, where some semblance of logical expectations – of ownership, of responsibility for actions – could be respected.

The futility behind so much of the anger unconsciously experienced by women patients seems to chase itself into similarly fruitless and unproductive, ultimately circular, directions. Tweenhood is the point at which social media begins to flex its adaptable fingers into the minds of ripely susceptible victims. Indeed, these platforms are expertly designed to capture and enthral a phase of brain development hungry for fast, candy-coloured fun, whilst insidiously urging those brains to identify in distorted ways with everything from 'unboxing' to filters. The endless accessibility and brilliantly personalised experience encourages Tween Girl to compare and covet and lose reality, trapping her further in a web of self-reproach and persecuted, obligatory feeling. A layering up of impotent, frustrated rage. Although Adult Women tell me they know what these constant feeds and reels are doing to them, somehow they can't back away. Their Tween brain is fully online. It's all about fitting in, standing out (the right amount), engendering envy, feeling the illusion of power. The addiction creates further disempowerment and loss of agency, which is disastrous for us women, who might better channel our energy into trying to claw up some substantial power IRL. The fear is that, if you stop imbibing the feed, you lose out. The potential to be involved escapes. We *know* these feelings from the playground. When a woman *does* appear to succeed in this world of spinning realities, she ultimately surrenders control to her own low self-esteem and lack of self-worth. A theme of not being able to win etches itself onto repeat, even in this made-up Monopoly universe, where 'followers' and 'likes' feel like genuine currency – the unwinnable popularity contest. From Tweens to Adult Women, we're just finding new ways to disempower ourselves.

I write at a time when the world seems poised on a precipice of chaos and dysregulation, so I'm not shocked that my clinic fills with women who feel existentially at sea – unmoored and unsecured since their own Tween years, having not been taught tools *then* which might have given them the confidence to say: 'Stop! I don't like this! I'm confused: what's happening?'

Instead, the swell of the current hurtles them forward into an unchartered ocean of expectation and demanding callousness, where the girl who one day is their BFF is tomorrow their frenemy, where segregation of the sexes means boys are no longer the equal playmates of yesterday. There's no safe harbour in adulthood either, no sequinned life raft to cling to here. The Adult Women versions of those Tweens come to me feeling betrayed by husbands who've shrunk away from emotionally matching them, leaving them to the swirling currents. Those men have floated off to their own life raft of work and sport (to which their own Tweens primed them) and left their wives to cope with the tedium. The rift between men and women is written back then in the Tween years, when society muscles in with its crass messaging and boring ideas about boys and girls.

The chat, intimacy and maturity encouraged and expected amongst Tween Girls is in opposition to the simplistic rough and tumble of boys' friendships. Predictably, this translates through to *wives'* phones filling with other mums' contact details, party invitations, dentist appointments and parents' evenings. Yes, maternity leave formalises this allocation of duties, but why does it perpetuate? In my view, those messages of Tween yesteryear embed the genderised experience of adulthood. The tenuous structure of 'team us', built on the desire and hormones of a few brief years of intensity, falls away. We look around for our teammate and ... er ... he's not taken up the position he promised to. The hard-won prize of equality doesn't *feel* equal. Our desire to Have It All can't compete with the reality of gender divisions in our past. That same lonely desire is now throttling us, leaving us gasping for air laced with SSRIs, melatonin and beta blockers.

Women conditioned into a sense of diminishment and playing it safe from Tweenhood seem stuck in a perpetual loop of lashing out at themselves. It's wrong to make a commotion or cause a stir. What if we embarrass him or hurt his feelings or make him feel humiliated? It starts with 'Be nice, Tweenie, don't *have it out with people.*' 'Don't be a nasty girl. Learn to bottle it and blame yourself.' 'Sit next to this "unruly" boy to exert your calming influence.'

WOMEN ARE <u>ANGRY</u>

Defeated and decimated, Tween Girl learns early to turn her own rage towards would-be female allies, projecting her more successful parts onto them and relating enviously with those projections. Later on, the overspill of unspent aggression and a sense of having failed lands on these other women, who provide the perfect hooks with their comparable attempts to juggle and make the impossible possible. It sounds like bitching. It is, in fact, psychic survival. Women, abandoned by their male counterparts, cling to whatever object they can to survive the onslaught of criticism and self-criticism thrown at them post-childbirth. Other women are often collateral damage. Where's the sisterhood when we need it most? It appears to turn against us as a weapon to assist the attack. Our Tweens are when that battle begins.

As we grow older, we continue to receive societal messages that our rage won't be tolerated as an overt phenomenon, which means we need to find other ways of releasing it. This may be as inversions, acts of harm against the self – from repression to actual physical trauma. Or as acts of passive aggression – forms of anger which have been disguised or semi-disguised to conceal their intended feeling; landing as confusing weapons of mass destruction, and lending the issuer the reputation of a manipulative or martyrish aggressor. But what are women to do? Unleash their fury wholesale, in no uncertain terms? Would that go down better?

The answer, I think, is to process the anger on a sort of rolling emotional conveyor belt so it doesn't have the chance to become stuck or calcified. When we attempt to express our needs in clearer and more straightforward ways, they're squeezed through a sort of wringer, stripped of some of their excess weight. In this way, they have the opportunity to hang in the air and receive their rightful hearing.

As an example, in my clinic I see many women who struggle to get on top of their anger. It's instead projected out onto me, often in spiteful and intolerable-feeling ways. When patients ask me to prepare statements about their experiences for legal or professional purposes, and I submit pieces which are, by necessity, constructed in the language of 'X has told me' rather than 'this is fact', these patients are invariably infuriated. At a personal level, I regret that I'm not able to say anything more categorical; I explain that I wasn't there, I'm not a witness to what happened. I'm a *therapist*, helping them to process the experience which they feel is theirs. That I am unable to write what they have reported to me as *fact* recreates the impotent rage dynamic that so often women are made to feel out there in the world and which has been there since those early Tween experiences, when girls learn that boys' voices are louder, that their boisterousness is tolerated and that less seems to be expected of them, emotionally. In short, the reality of their being heard and taken seriously feels remote.

At least when such a sense of loss and betrayal arrives in therapy, we're able to work it through together, via the painful yet informative transference experience. They have an opportunity to tell another woman *to her face* what it feels like that she's let them down. That she's betrayed their trust. This is something that we were robbed of in those Tween years, when society decreed that we had to get a mutual friend to tell our BFF we weren't talking to her.

In this way, the patient can instead come to practise what it is to know the pattern, know the root of the pattern and choose to operate differently in future. By taking umbrage with the therapist for the cards society's stacked against her, deeper exploration of the anger this incites is invited by the therapist, and both parties come to understand the primitive buttons which are pressed: the childhood abandonment or neglect or parental failure to hear and see; the teacher's lack of time or resources to be able to sit with Tween Girls and help them work out more honest, direct ways of communicating, so they didn't have to rely on the backstab and bitching. Society has stoked this, in its stirring up of envy and competition, so that, by the point she's in therapy, the female patient is so far from what she may have identified as anger, so worn down and resigned, that it's easier to treat the stomach problems or the unforgiving headaches which have instead risen up as symptoms following any kind of conflictual encounter with a colleague or friend.

By finally engaging with a relationship which encourages contact with the cause of the issue, she's given permission to connect with and take responsibility for her pain. She can find a different voice, a stronger voice, which bypasses the irritable passivity borne of feeling impeded. She can tap into what she really feels hurt by, and name it. She can say to me, as her therapist, 'I'm really angry and hurt that, after all the hours you've spent appearing to hear my story and take it seriously, you throw me under the bus with this anodyne piece of shit letter. Which, by its very omissions, seems to suggest I'm nuts. I feel gaslit and betrayed.'

Finally, in a relationship she can trust and, with someone who looks like they can take it, she can scream and rail and mourn what she hasn't had, until there's enough room to be able to see what she *does* have – and knit all of these strengths together under the unconditional gaze of her therapist (that important, unbroken gaze again) who will encourage her to boldly test out this new set of strengths and unleash the voice it gives rise to. She will be encouraged to use it out there, in the world, with people who – much to her surprise – are suddenly more inclined to hear her. Now that she's finally being listened to, properly heard after all these years, the anger subsides. Her stomach problems ease, she notices fewer headaches. Fewer experiences of conflict arise because she can express the feelings she now has a bolder, cleaner pipeline down into.

I can't be your therapist in real life, but I can show you to how to look deeper into your own experiences. I can remind you how much crap is set up for us from such a young age. And how, as adults, we need to remember to parent that child within us, who almost certainly didn't get the robust messages she needed back then to set her up for experiences of equality now. Let these examples of other women like you help show how different things can be.

Billie
Anger as resentment. Her strategy = Get her life back

Billie had been a very good Tween Girl. She was now married to a man whose career was his identity. The teaching she'd received from her religious family of origin was that Little Girls would be quiet and mild-mannered and angelic. Billie hadn't invested in friendships since her

Tweens, when a group of supposed friends scapegoated and ostracised her. Because she'd been gagged by the strictness of her upbringing, Billie wasn't in a position to defend herself against these girls' behaviours, nor to see the behaviours as necessarily problematic. Billie simply accepted the meanness as somehow correctly intentioned. She didn't understand what she'd done wrong, but knew she must have done *something* wrong. It simply never occurred to her that these bullies might have been the wrongdoers.

Now an adult, the assumption was that, after having their three children, she would give up her career as a flight attendant (another example of how easily Billie could be pushed around). Because she'd had babies across the pandemic years, support had been negligible and she wasn't able to form any female connections then either. Her husband was wrapped up in his professional pursuits, now that the onus was on him to earn (his ambitions had been less than practical, and always more about actualisation and personal fulfilment).

As resentment and lack of understanding grew between them, Billie began to feel increasingly lonely and isolated. This seemed to irk her husband, who saw her sadness as controlling and needy. She would cry that his inability to see beyond his own desires was a barrier to understanding her predicament. He levelled back that she was 'gaslighting him'. (You wouldn't believe how much this term is wrongly used, mostly by the gaslighter themselves.) His defensiveness was instant whenever she mentioned the reality of being at home caring for tiny children. He'd distort that reality, and argue he'd never asked for a life which involved being apart from his children. And that *he* was busy 'earning money to care for them all' (this was barely true).

So often, Adult Women seem to be up against the argument of, 'I'm doing this for you, for the family.' Even Billie didn't have a leg to stand on here, especially when money was flung into the mix and he referenced the material things his money had paid for ... a cheap, odious shot when she has no choice but to be at home with their children. Though, if she'd been working, she'd have brought home twice the amount he was bringing in. I'm struck by the number of women returning to work after maternity leave, who pronounce that their paid job is several times easier than being at home doing the childcare had been. And by how many of their male partners insist on upholding the myth that *they* have the raw deal because they 'never had that time at home'.

What I've noticed in my practice is that a number of male partners seem to have to furiously peddle the narrative that they're hard done by, that they're the ones truly suffering. This mantra grows more feverish the more women are eventually reminded that, actually, the world of work is infinitely less demanding than being at home with the thankless load. In some instances, this gets really nasty. I've seen more or less conscious attempts to really bring a woman down, Hitchcock-style. Doubt is poured on her mental health and psychological stability to the extent that she doubts herself, begins to wonder if she does indeed have **PND** or possibly 'borderline personality disorder', and accepts that *she*'s the weak one for struggling with the task most of her husband's friends' wives have 'no problem with'. If our Tweens hadn't primed us for the role of being excellent and capable, as well as absolutely *conforming*, we might have had better grounding in when to scream, 'This situation is mad, I'm not standing for it and it's not *my* failure!'

There still seems to be a tendency to eulogise and place on a pedestal the women who appear to be serenely coping, with no nod to the probable unravelling behind the scenes. Remember the Tween Girl asked to placate the dysregulated boy? The Tween Girl roped in to entertain babies or write lovely 'thank you' cards? Or sit quietly in her meagre square of playground and chat? Though 'chat' can mean 'bitchy attack', it can also mean relational richness. We connect. We find companionship, support and kinship.

Billie needed friends. Obviously, her Tweens had scarred her. Those cruel behaviours girls feel they've no choice but to identify with haunted her into adulthood, when she needed other women and the bolstering of shared experience more than ever before. I prescribed playgroups, coffee mornings, nights out with mums. Screw that it's become a cliché. These communities exist for a reason. People who don't have much power can at least band together and feel seen and known. I urged

Billie to be honest and share her feelings, to really open herself to forge connections. Over time, Billie began to dare to trust other women (starting with trusting me, her therapist). She began to build these relationships, meet allies and find strength and independence. She's now working on occasional flights again. Her husband is still flapping about with his career and has missed out on a lot of his opportunity to parent. Sad, but true. Come on, boys: help us out here!

As I mentioned, working with an individual provides inevitable indirect access to other family members. Sometimes, when a partner figuratively forces their way repeatedly into a therapy treatment, you have to wonder: why do they have to occupy so much of our session time? Why can't they leave us alone? We spent so long talking about Billie's husband's career choice and neuroses that I felt he should probably get his own issues looked at (I mean, who shouldn't anyway?). It just feels rude to use someone else's therapy for it. I find it's when male partners are too frightened to enter into their own therapeutic work that they come crashing into our space.

I've noticed an established pattern of men using their female partners as therapists – frequently flagrantly admitting so. But often, their problems are so overwhelming that a woman can't carry them by herself. However, the session hijack is also because women avoid giving themselves the opportunity to really take the consulting room for themselves. It feels intimidating to be given that permission. We've never been encouraged. What we've learnt is: sit still, be nice, if you have an issue with someone, talk about it behind their back.

For children coming into the consulting room via a parent, it's a different matter. This is partially because so many of our own issues get played out through our parenting, so often their stuff *is* our stuff. Also because it really does take a village to raise a child, and therapists are well placed to help you think about what's going on for the kid who isn't in the room. And to lend a containing and thoughtful space to reflect on what might be happening in the relationship. This was the case for Angel and her Tween Girl Mishka.

Mishka
Anger as muteness. Her strategy = Martial arts

Mishka was ten and highly anxious. She cried every morning before school and had one friend who sometimes refused to talk to her and played with other girls instead. Angel would weep with helplessness about her daughter, and talked about how Mishka had even started to have panic attacks on a Sunday night, where she felt unable to breathe and as if her heart was 'beating too fast'. Mishka thought she was dying in these distressing moments, and Angel struggled to comfort her. Angel was a single mum, with a demanding job and a very supportive same-sex partner who didn't live with them, but who helped care for Mishka and was a solid pillar in her life. Both women felt completely lost about what to do with this poor little girl who had apparently always been reserved, but who now was disappearing in front of them.

A few weeks into my work with Angel, Mishka became mute. Angel flew into understandable panic and needed a lot of containment. Angel's partner, Tia, and I seemed to form an unofficial alliance around Angel, and we almost parented her through her own collapse, so that she could remain consistent towards Mishka.

Whilst Mishka was placed on a never-ending waiting list for state psychological support, I knew we needed to take speedy action, for Angel's sake as well as her daughter's. One incredible thing to remember about children, though, is that their brains are so adaptive that, when they bounce back (which can happen really quickly), they can get themselves to a place which feels unrecognisable. You'll have seen this when kids are ill physically – their health really can transform practically overnight.

It's the same for psychological suffering. We need to ascertain the best treatment – sometimes watchful waiting (as with physical illness), sometimes gentle intervention and, in some cases, therapy. But we then need to let them become well; we need to allow the bounceback, the recovery, the freedom from labels. Otherwise the 'anxious child' becomes the 'anxious adult' and the self-limiting human and the 'anxious parent' – and so the cycle persists.

Because of the urgency here, I took a more firmly practical hand than usual and helped Angel think about a physical, social type of 'explosive' exercise close to their home. She found a martial arts centre which offered mixed classes to pre-teen children. Mishka was obviously reticent, but both Angel and Tia promised to wait outside whilst she went to her first karate class. Apparently, she stood silently at the back and didn't involve herself, but the instructor was adept at dealing with any eventuality and took it in his stride. She didn't make a big deal of it and, over weeks, became a very calm, very reliable older female presence in Mishka's life. The summer holidays approached and, though Mishka still wasn't speaking at school, she asked Angel to sign her up for the holiday karate club with Femi, the female instructor.

Angel was pretty astounded, but, of course, took her along, with plenty of assurances that she could pick her up early and that it was fine for her to change her mind about going (to Tia's and – privately – my own frustration, since she threatened to put Mishka off). But Mishka went. And something happened across that week – something huge. Mishka made two new friends. Both boys. Both wonderful, beautiful boys. The best of tween males. Non-judgemental, straightforward, funny, cheeky, playful. Really playful. And cheerfully boisterous, which seemed to allow Mishka to find her aggression and channel it outwards – we all have it in us.

Brought up amongst women, however intuitive and warm and intelligent this parenting had been, her childhood hadn't been rambunctious. And Mishka had anger in her. A particular kid in her class had been targeting Mishka for not having a dad. Although there'd been open conversation around her IVF conception, and

Mishka's feelings had been discussed and understood as far as possible by Angel and Tia, the world comes in with all of its cruelty and prejudice. Whilst we can't protect them entirely, perhaps we can help our Tween Girls to at least register their feelings about this somewhere which isn't their own body.

I think at this age, between childhood and not-quite adolescence, we're especially vulnerable to feelings of displacement and confusion. Such feelings can overtake us before we have an opportunity to know what they're about or really be able to recognise them. For Mishka, school dynamics and other children's words had also contributed to her overwhelm. Of course, it wasn't all plain sailing from there – life just isn't – but Mishka emerged from that particular experience without a label, and Angel could come back to therapy for herself. This case illustrates how much women can offer each other. As well as how joyful and constructive the experiences between male and female can be.

What we can do for Tween Girl

As we've seen, the Tween years are where behavioural difference and social treatment really begin to tell at the level of gender. We can all try to address the habits we've formed around kids of this age by:

- Encouraging play between sexes.

- Partnering kids of opposite sexes in school and other activities.
- Encouraging a range of play styles.
- Trying to keep things like birthday parties mixed.
- In these 'latency' years, boys are often seen as emotionally incapable, so girls can feel more powerful and sophisticated. But this is where the problem begins. We shouldn't exploit this apparent capability by adulting Tween Girl.
- Nor should we allow boys to get away with behaviour they could actually attend to and evolve within. Let's not create emotionally limited men. If they learn to expand themselves now, it sets up a foundation for later life and better intersex relationships.
- Let's get boys and girls talking together about what's happening, about what's on each other's mind. Let's create a mind which isn't so binary and gendered. Let's get them really listening to each other.
- Encourage girls to see their bodies as their own strong, healthy possession.
- Look at the way our own Tweenhood may have set us up for particular patterns in adulthood. It's never too late to challenge these assumptions in ourselves. Why are we always the fixers, the sorters, the planners? Step back!

Scrape off those glittery tattoos and grab some pimple patches. We're heading into the world of adolescence proper …

CHAPTER SEVEN

Teen Girl

THE TEEN YEARS can be tough for anyone. But, for girls, the stats are skewed. From eating disorders to self-harm to body dysmorphia, it's a potential minefield. Nowadays, it's obviously all played out on the public, permanent, painful platform of social media. Being a Teen Boy is no walk in the park, but that's a whole other book. Here, we explore the psychology of developing within a woman's body.

Our bodies are ultimately the playground and battlefield on which so much of society enforces its envious regulation. The complex chemical events initiating Teenhood kick off the tendency for our own physical scaffolding to result in feelings of anger internally, in the form of menstrual rage. But Teen Girl also comes to know the capacity of her body to incite the frightened fury of those intimidated by its potential.

As women, we have a hole within us, in the form of a uterus which can be filled with the most potent possibility of all – a baby. But this makes us vulnerable to exploitation, male envy and a need for them to fearfully occupy and own us. Just as male animals might eat their offspring, the potential we possess for popping out an object which might overpower them one day is unconsciously threatening to some.

The rage emanating from inside and outside of us is ultimately absorbed and contained within ourselves. All children are vulnerable, but as soon as a girl develops breasts, she comes to know a different, lifelong fear. In synchrony with her literal bursting out of her too-tight skin, men are lusting after her clueless body. Women patients refer to the Teen years as the point at which they began to feel the punishing cage of their female body, in which self-disgust and vulnerability met with the cruel ogling of the outside world.

This chapter explores the power and impotency of what it is to be born into a woman's body, the ways our brain has already been co-opted to internalise the frustrations of this and how we can create a different relationship with our physical selves.

Let's begin by thinking about the structure of desire. The male gaze has a lot to answer for when it comes to women's anger. We've been heavily indoctrinated to view a man pinning us in his sights as something to feel grateful for and excited about. This deeply conditioned response is so overwhelming that we're not easily able to disentangle or define our own intuition or desire. I think this is why so many women I see feel confused about the relationships and sexual experiences they've had, which have left them unsatisfied or denigrated. The increasing recognition of 'rude not to' encounters as unacceptable had the potential to bring a sea change. Based on what I hear in clinic, it hasn't. Women of all ages are still left questioning what they've consented to, and how entitled they are to voice their doubts. From 2016, there has been a 'catastrophic decline in rape prosecutions' according to The Victims Commissioner. Society is sending the message it doesn't know how to support us. The pressure towards politeness and obligation can trump whether or not, as a woman, you feel you've really agreed to something. Which is where the necessity to be good, to be nice, to be kind, to be thoughtful as Little Girl and Tween Girl really stitches us up.

Naming assaultive behaviour as such can be alarming to women, particularly if they're younger and haven't yet begun to stand in scrutiny of what they've been socialised to accept. Sadly, women who've come to me for support in recovering from a case they've identified as assault and attempted to take further frequently find themselves victim to a double attack. They're forced to relive the experience again and again, and are themselves held to account and scrutinised. These double blows do appear to be a universal feature of feminine experience. You try to take a stand, to raise your voice, to tell your story, but doing so within a system geared to silence and oppress invariably leaves you worse off.

The way in which my female patients have felt themselves to be in servitude to male desire since their earliest teens aligns with many other ways in which their later roles are defined. The inequities between men and women find parallel form and wrap around each other, so that apparently unrelated predicaments end up merged. The pseudo-servitude of female childhood – being well-behaved and neat and clean and helpful – morphs into the servitude of appeasing the male gaze, which morphs into the later assumptions around our domestic life. Which, in turn, inhibits our professional ambitions and confidence.

The way we see ourselves becomes entirely defined by others – if not by men *per se*, certainly those structures established within a patriarchy. Structures which best serve the people who dreamt them up.

And so our anger grows. And grows. As the potential for abuses of power in this way *increases* rather than *decreases* throughout our lives, the anger that pulses forth has fewer outlets. Our plight feels more inevitable. The anger can only be internalised. Another migraine. A panic attack. Worsening IBS. High blood pressure. Cancer.

Perversely, I've noticed that a woman can actually feel furious with a man, but that this anger, claimed and distorted by the male gaze, can translate back to the woman as attraction. Sure, she's got some powerful emotions circulating. Society tells her this is 'sexual tension', this is frenzied, inhibited desire. Romcoms are structured around the idea of a woman feeling infuriated with, or even disgusted by, a man, only to somehow 'learn' that what she really feels is a deep attraction to him. Through this lens, we can see how diminishing and denigrating this narrative is to her emotions.

An 18-year-old patient described the following incident, a real-life consequence of our indoctrination into feeling we have few choices. She was on the London Underground, travelling to work very early. On the platform, she was alone with a man who suddenly started walking towards her very quickly. She thought, 'He'll just be walking past, he's realised he's on the wrong platform.' But he walked right up to her, ravishing a burger, quite incongruously, and stared into her face. This wasn't funny. This was horrible. She was between the man and the track. She ducked and walked at pace away from him, down the steps, hoping she'd soon bump into another person. She didn't. She had to go all the way back to the ticket hall, as she just didn't feel safe in this maze of passages, alone with a man. She told herself – but there are cameras everywhere! Its 7am on a weekday morning – what can happen? But in that precise moment, she was alone. No one was coming to help her. She was entirely vulnerable. When she emerged from underground, she felt so shaken up that she wasn't able to make contact with her rage for some time – until her session two days later, in fact.

What she then pieced together was: a man had invaded her space and made her feel threatened – which had made her late for her day, for the job she loves and was minding her own business to honour. But at that time, trapped in an underground labyrinth, she just felt fear. This wasn't newsworthy though, was it? It was completely run of the mill and unreportable. You'll all have had countless similar experiences. What would she have said to another (probably male) Underground attendant? 'A man charged up to me on the platform, chomping on a burger?' She'd be laughed at, and would have then been even later for her day. And, thus, it goes on ... Another banal, shitty, psychologically damaging incident in a Young Woman's life.

A separate public transport incident concerning a different young patient involved aggressive staring. Again, a quiet Tube carriage at the same time of day; not empty, but no one else noticed. The thread of unbroken threat flowing from the man opposite her was invisible to everyone else. As with the previous patient, anger was not the emotion which arrived easily. She felt first humiliated. She squirmed. She felt disgusted. She felt she must be doing something to invite his gaze. Her expression had been too inviting and friendly when she first clocked him. She told me later, 'I shouldn't have smiled.' Where was her anger? Converted into a flavour of fearful, inverted rage which acts upon the self, instead of radiating outwards, towards the target.

The consulting room fills with myriad unremarkable tales of daily disturbance. It's so boring and so usual, we find a mental shorthand for it. We learn from very young to avoid the male gaze, to not be alone in a train carriage, to perfect the art of covering up our bodies with our bodies. But these are microaggressions; tedious, run-of-the-mill microaggressions, which begin here and end up sitting inside of us. The disgusted, suppressed rage we feel has to go somewhere. It's energy; it doesn't disappear. We ultimately absorb it. And these Teen years are spent perfecting the art.

Alternatively, we may think we have a handle on it. In a sense, this could appear to be a kind of female power at play. She unconsciously selects to override her natural feeling state (grossed out), and converts the disempowerment into something positive. She has the upper hand, because this is a sort of choice. *Is* this a sort of deep, knowing certainty, in which women have a goddess-like superiority and are the ones in control all along? It could indeed be the basis on which so much of the oppression we face is built – a terror in men that we really are the clever ones, the seducers, the bearers of power. The iron girders which contain us need therefore to be stronger than ever. The more potent women become, in equal and opposite force the bars of the cage around them must squeeze.

Even if this is the case, those cage bars pinch and twist and bruise our flesh. Women talk a lot in the consulting room about the pain of coming into their bodies as Teen Girl; about realising the ownership that society has over them. Everyone recalls the first leering looks, the envious, lascivious gaze emanating from men and women alike – the women themselves loaded up with their own complex feelings towards femininity and power. My patients speak of the exposing nature of this protracted and shaming experience; the felt vulgarity of their uncontrollable bodies; the sense of debasement as they squirmed beneath the weight of lust, expectation and pressure that this body represented for others: 'I didn't own myself', 'I loathed being inside of my own skin', 'I felt I was spilling out everywhere', 'Everything about me that was most private was public.'

This is the age when we experience the terror of being at school or in public and finding that our tampon or pad has leaked. It is when we sit exams whilst feeling sick, faint or even anaemic, with a vicelike headache and crippling abdominal cramps. This is the age where we learn to give the colour white a very wide berth, from trousers to sofas to bedding. Of course, boys have their issues at this age, but without the baked-in monthly dread that their bodies could feasibly let them down in a way that could be catastrophic to their future selves, socially and academically. But for God's sake, don't mention it. Start perfecting the tampon-up-sleeve, back to the wall shuffle, then tear up the corridor. One patient recounted how, when she was a Teen Girl and on her period on a long family car journey, her dad made such a fuss about stopping for a break that she had to sit on a magazine to ensure she wouldn't bleed through to the seat. Her brothers were oblivious, such was their privilege.

As we try to grow up with some sense of a solid identity, one which is ours and we've chosen for ourselves, we navigate not only the overt ogling and denigration, but also that which comes from so-called 'feminist men' who pretend to support us. Even 'We love the natural look!' or 'Just be yourself!' become ways of insidiously giving out instructions, laying down demands, 'allowing' us to try out a different Barbie dress-up. Our looks are policed and patrolled, so that gaining a real sense of who we are underneath the glare of the patriarchal gaze becomes a remote possibility. On this note, let's meet Toya, whose teenhood had been forged within the furnace of the ultra-internalised patriarchy: the all-girl private school.

Toya
Anger as fragile superiority and self-harm.
Her strategy = Yoga and punching

Why is it that we don't have an equivalent label for Boarding School Syndrome (the trauma of being sent to boarding school at a very young age, often the domain of emotionally cauterised men) for the epidemic of psychological issues we see stemming from girls' private schools? Whilst Boarding School Syndrome is real and horrible, there's also a phenomenon affecting girls at elite private schools which we don't discuss as much. We know it's a thing, we know that eating disorders and self-harm are rife at these institutions, but why doesn't this have a name? It can't be because the privilege turns us away from labelling, as we have a name for the boarding school issue, and you could argue nothing is posher than this. Is it because it only affects girls?

TEEN GIRL

Girls and women tend, again, to internalise their frozen anger and pain about experiences which eat away at their ability to control. We know that this can frequently present in the form of eating disorders and self-harm. These are acts of violence against the self which are tucked inside and which don't get an opportunity for airing, unless the victim can identify her feelings as stemming from rage and a deep sense of anguished injustice, and find a healthier release. This is what (eventually) happened for Toya.

Toya had been sent to a traditional girls' school as a young teen by her parents, who were from outside the UK and had fetishised the importance of an elite English education. Toya came to see me in her late twenties, desperate to please and to let me know that I'd said the right thing, whilst also feeling very brittle and hard to reach. Her accent was cut-glass and there was a primness to her which seemed to communicate disapproval. She *appeared* to project her anger by letting the other person know she found them inferior, which, it emerged, was in fact her own feeling. This superior/inferior tension was the locus around which her rage tried to work its way out with circular, self-punishing results.

Since being Teen Girl, Toya had been plagued by the sensation that people found her inconsequential. Her defence was managing to make *them* feel it by creating distance and difficulty in her relationships, which were mostly held at arms' length. You can see why one refuge for a Teen Girl would be locked away inside of herself, hidden from the frenzy of projections coming at her like meteors. The trouble is, when we furiously lock ourselves away, we lock ourselves down. It's global. We get further away from everyone, including ourselves. In trying to shield ourselves from feeling, we numb ourselves to experience. We don't give ourselves a chance to feel the outside world isn't a threat, and we don't find out that our own feelings can be tolerated. In order to give herself a moderated, controlled experience of her rage, Toya had deeply sliced up the top of her thighs with a knife, the scars etching a roadmap of her agony. 'All the girls did it. It was normal.'

Tolerating my proximity and potential threat became our first goal. Out in the world, I suggested activities which connected Toya to her body and externalised her rage, in a way that she could feel in control of. She chose yoga, because it seemed safe and predictable. After a few months, she reported that she'd had to stop because she would cry her way through a class. We discussed why she felt this to be a problem. She looked appalled: 'Adults don't cry!'

I wondered aloud whether a punchbag to hang in her back garden could ever be appealing to Toya. A couple of months later, she told me that she'd actually bought one straight away. But another device she had for keeping me away from her was through a kind of cagey secrecy. What she now revealed was that she'd begun to balance punching with yoga (which she had taken up again, but still only did privately, because of the crying). This mix of release, of punching out her raw Teen rage and crying out the pain, seemed to connect her to her feelings in ways which then enabled a deeper interplay between us in the therapy room. As she began to feel herself as more human, she made me feel less chaotic and outré. I took this as a sign she'd also begun to allow for more real feelings in herself. She no longer had to present as the put-together automaton. The brutal teachings of Teenhood, the severing of herself from her own emotional core, had meant that recalibrating was required to enable a healthier connection with herself and others. She needed to first get rid of the oceans of rage and discharge them physically, before she could find space and tolerance for the more connected experiences of yoga and therapy.

I'll introduce you now to Nyra, whose teens had also marked the beginning of derailment.

Nyra
Anger as generalised anxiety. Her strategy = Separating thoughts from feelings

Nyra was in her early thirties when she came to see me. Since being a teenager, she'd suffered with generalised anxiety, social anxiety and intrusive obsessive thoughts. She was a teacher, but felt as if she was hanging on to her profession by the skin of her teeth, and that all her friends had better strategies than her for managing their careers.

She looked at the systems they seemed to put in place for handling their workload, and imagined that the success she saw them enjoy followed as a direct result of that. Because her emotional reserves felt so compromised, she cast about and found ways to punish herself by focusing on the perceived skill of others.

Since being a Teen Girl, Nyra had also experienced frequent intrusive thoughts concerning the safety of her parents. She imagined their involvement in horrific accidents, and was always frightened to ask what they were up to, in case they told her they were planning a trip in the car. Based on the psychoanalytic idea of wish fulfilment, we might deduce a certain fantasy around her parents' death. Because stating that aloud would have sent Nyra running a mile, I gently suggested instead that, underneath anxiety, we often find a surprising amount of anger, which she dubiously accepted as a concept. This allowed us to get to work.

First off, I wanted to get on top of the life-inhibiting symptoms that were torturing Nyra to such an extent that she feared for her job, her friendships and her new partnership. Although contentious for many traditionally psychoanalytic therapists, my view is: we need to be realistic. We need to help people live in the real world and get them back on track as quickly as possible – we need to enable them to regain strength to do the deep digging safely. Without doubt, it's the deep dig which will safeguard patients from repeat episodes, but we need to first build a bedrock of resilience before this can get going. So we stick on the temporary Band-Aid whilst the work shapes out underneath.

For Nyra, this meant getting a handle on her repetitive, self-destructive thoughts. I encouraged her to become a sleuth with her own mental processes. She started to recognise her anxious thoughts forming from further away. Her neck would prickle 'almost electrically'. Her heart rate would increase, her breathing grow fast and shallow. I encouraged her to focus on identifying whether these physiological events follow a thought or whether the thought surfaces almost to *explain* the physical symptom. By concentrating hard on the symptoms as they arose, Nyra discovered that, initially, her body would start sending these signals 'out of nowhere'. Her mind would then cast about looking for the reason. Because the thought patterns of 'something terrible is going to happen to my parents' and 'I'm losing my grip' seemed indelible, they became containers; familiar ruts to channel the feeling into. Once she began to scrutinise them in this way, the individuated feelings started to feel more like ports which were adequate for storing the affect, rather than arriving as a result of it.

As Nyra's thoughts began to clarify, they were more available for scrutiny. Where had they come from? What did they articulate? We had the fears about life rejecting her; we had the fears about her parents rejecting her (albeit via 'accident'). Once Nyra had recognised that the thought followed the feeling, she could block the thought as it arose and attend to the feeling. I taught her some basic breathing exercises, which she tried to practise on the hour. Any thoughts which threatened to tip her back into the feeling she'd compile in a phone note which she brought in to me. In this way, she evacuated them from her mind and waited to show them to mine. Together, we'd look at what she'd recorded.

Nyra gradually arrived into a more regulated state. This meant we were able to turn our attention to *why* the angry feeling (I insisted on calling it this, as opposed to anxiety) and why these particular thoughts arose. From this now calmer state began our more typical psychoanalytic journey through the annals of her unconscious. We discovered that her parents, so torn up and furious at their own dismal experience of being parented, had resolved their pain through being negligent towards their own daughter. In her teens, they really cut her loose. They were detached from her internal world and the objects in it, including friends and school. Nyra was expected to take care of herself, emotionally. She didn't make a fuss about this (what was the point?); instead, she got on with it, patching together an internal scaffolding for herself and doing her best to adapt it to her changing needs. I hear this a lot – Teen Girl looks so convincingly together and mature, even kind parents can make the mistake of leaving them to it. Teen Girl behaviours can seem rejecting in response to this (as with Toya), which can really exacerbate the loop.

When Nyra was 14, her mum left her and her dad and went to live in a neighbouring town. Although Nyra saw her at weekends, she ended up mothering *her* during these visits, rather than the other way around. Her mother became more and more isolated, and angry in her isolation. Nyra's arrival into her Teen Girl body threatened her mum. The potential of Nyra's womanhood was experienced as a kind of taunt. Nyra's mum felt that those years were lost to her now, and her daughter's potential was felt as an attack. Nyra's dad, in a pointed and self-righteous way, coupled up with another woman. But Nyra, the dutiful Teen Girl, allowed herself to bear the brunt of her mother's wrath and her father's rejection. She didn't complain; she saw it as her due. Because this is how, as young women, we're conditioned to respond to others' needs.

Nyra began to be aware of how envious she herself had felt towards the friends who, in her fantasy, had been the recipients of nourishing home lives; one which had seemed to lead to a position of richness over their choices and careers. This atmosphere of envy and self-diminishment, of angry deprivation, had permeated her mother's life and was beginning to permeate her own. Though Nyra had been forced to put up such a strong front of not needing her parents, she nonetheless smarted psychologically at their cruel and deliberate-seeming rejection. All previous narratives defending their actions were clearly designed to protect her from the reality that they'd behaved so hatefully towards her. The ego wound of this humiliation required a good deal of defending from – a use of energy which no doubt increased the levels of unconscious rage within her, channelled more conveniently into feelings of anxiety, designed to further silence the self. Even Nyra's relationship with her girlfriend Hannah had been suffering. Hannah's family seemed to represent the epitome of capability and support, and what they'd given Hannah appeared to have set her up in life. Another source of rage in Nyra, as she found increasing trust in our relationship and could speak more freely, stemmed from the envy she was experiencing in a passive way by witnessing Hannah's very different confidence levels.

The commonality between Nyra's experience and that of so many other women I've worked with is the apparent *acceptance* of her lot. Just like her mother before her, there was no outward display of the rage and sense of injustice she harboured. Her mother, the more disenfranchised and wounded by life she felt, would *appear* to inflict the pain upon herself. But the sharp whip-end of this rancour also cut Nyra. As Nyra's mother constructed a life which looked increasingly lonely and embittered, she'd (consciously or unconsciously) created suffering in her teenage daughter. The mother's disavowal of her own anger meant that it lurked like a shark in the gap between her and her daughter. Dumping her anger into this place, from where it nipped at Nyra when it felt like it, provided some form of respite for her mum. This must have only been temporary – which is why it had to run on repeat.

Because Nyra was initially unable to see the treatment from her mum as hateful – because why would a mother place hate on her child? That's too disgustingly painful – it became easier to split the feeling. She began to part-project it onto others, in an envious form, and part-relate to it as 'anxiety' within herself. After all, in this day and age, who *doesn't* suffer with anxiety?

Following the identification of these processes, Nyra began to 'forget' about her symptoms. This isn't the same thing as 'curing', because actually her brain just needed to be shown another path to follow. Nyra one day piped up, 'You know, I think I actually *wanted* Mum and Dad dead! It feels like my worry about something happening to them was more of a fantasy than a fear, now I've come to think about it ...'

The objective analysis of her thoughts helped to condition Nyra's mind away from the tendency to fall into that particular groove, whilst the identification of the deeper mechanism beneath the behaviours established a scaffold of rational explanation which soothed Nyra's pain and strengthened her internally. Some of the areas of deficit and confusion are bolstered by this retrospective binding. There is, over time, a sense that the 'search is over' and that the losses of childhood no longer need to define the present.

The way I visually explain the success of this approach is as follows: identifying the missing 'bars' in one's internal scaffolding and simultaneously providing the experience of being held in an infantile way is the equivalent of going back into the past and roping together the missing parts. These may never be as strong as they would have been if they'd been provided by our primary carers – they may always be our psychic weak spots –

but if we're aware of them, and can top up with help for that as we develop through our lives, we can avoid the gap widening and threatening the entire structure. Equally, neurons which fire together wire together, so if we keep practising these newly self-aware modes of behaving, ensuring that we make the best use of new pathways, reminding ourselves what we're doing and why, there's no reason why these pathways can't become as established and solid as any other.

Here, I can try to draw women's attention to the ways in which they internalise anger, and how harmful to their minds, bodies and relationships this is. I think, given a bit of honest self-talk, we can all go some way to helping ourselves identify areas of pain. Through simple behavioural methods like thought analysis, note-taking and breathwork, we can, to some extent, become our own therapists. Through exercise and screaming and punching things, we can alleviate a lot of internal anguish. But, most of all, we need to learn to communicate. Therapy is without doubt the best way of working through uncomfortable or stuck dynamics, but the next best thing is to create transparent connections with those around us.

We need to learn to talk to each other in ways which most directly communicate our needs, and which are most open to hearing the needs of others in return. We need to talk about hatred and rage and terror, even if it feels like they shouldn't fit in polite society. When we can call things what they actually are, we free ourselves from some of the feeling they leave in us.

We need to learn to depend on trusted friends, colleagues and relatives, and begin building better connections with them. When we haven't had parents we can rely on, this can be a challenge. What we've also started to see from the stories here are the ways in which our conditioning continues to inform us across diverse levels. For instance, having a disinterested, uninvolved dad sets you up for expecting little from an adult male partner. If we decide we're going the other way, and choose a man who does support us properly, we have to work against ourselves and our wiring. Rewriting the past can feel exhausting.

But we can begin to form different habits in small ways which yield significant results. Even framing what we say in simple terms of 'I feel' or 'This makes me feel', rather than anything more defensive, spiky or passive. Being straight-forwardly truthful quickly alerts others to our willingness to be vulnerable, and encourages expression of their vulnerability in return. We need to be able to tolerate displays of emotion better – even in the workplace. Men and women need to be able to cry, to talk about hurt and pain and feeling poorly treated. Katya was a good example of someone who found expressing her negative feelings extremely difficult. Let's hear her story.

Katya
Anger as brittle hatred. Her strategy = Talking and crying

Katya was furiously trying to be the right thing in an industry which wasn't making room for her anymore. She came to see me as a buttoned-up, gagged 43-year-old. She had worked in fashion since she arrived in the UK in her twenties. She felt she was 'getting too old' and that people were passing her over and phasing her out. The brittleness this incited in her was palpable, and entered the room. She was often picking up on faults in me and pointed out my wrongdoings mercilessly. Working with her was initially horrible and I had to frequently fight the instinct to walk away.

Her dad had died when she was a teenager and Katya was livid. She'd already been raging in the way Teen Girl needs to, when her father became ill with an aggressively degenerative illness. What you *don't* want in the midst of a Teen rage is for that parent to die. Katya remained forever frozen in her guilt-ridden fury, further encumbered by an anger that her dad had now actually abandoned her. The tightly packed-in layers of toxic feeling seemed absolutely represented by Katya's current ground-in presentation and viciously passive behaviours.

Katya needed help to find her voice, let alone her anger. As well as in our sessions together, I encouraged her to *talk talk talk* outside in the world; to overspeak, to overexpress, to overshare. Her 'too much' was most people's ordinary. When we talk, we process. To process feelings of rage is to free ourselves and be able to live a life unhampered by the internal pain they cause. I not only encouraged her to speak, but to shout. To holler. To roar loudly in the shower. To yell her aggression into cushions or pillows. To yell her head off in the car. To shriek onto motorways from bridges high up, where no one could hear her and the wind would carry away her pain. If we hadn't been in London, I'd have encouraged clifftop or hilltop shouting too. But this approach had to be modified for urban, clustered dwelling.

Gradually, Katya began to cry and soften and grieve. Her hard edges melted, her friendships deepened and job opportunities came along. The traumatised rage of her Teen Girl years had merged with the impotent anger she experienced as an adult, in a world which threatened her with abandonment once again. By identifying the anger, past and present, we enabled Katya to channel the power of that inverted energy and use it to navigate sexist systemic structures with a new and confident zeal. She was now a woman, not a furiously agonised child. Her anger was available to her and could be appropriately mobilised to achieve her goals in a sector typically hostile to women of a certain age.

Teen Girl is forced to realise that her biology has reverberating repercussions across her life which boys know no equivalent to. One of the ways this plays out concerns the issue of contraception. Any sexually active woman will at some point have come up against the realisation that, when it comes to contraceptive medicine, *listed side effects* mean something. For my patient, Nina, her daughter Kezzia's early contact with the combined contraceptive pill ushered in an eating disorder – a fact which deeply rankles with the feminist in me. The pill was meant to be the answer! It was meant to spell our liberation! In significant ways, it has, but the larger reality around this pseudo-liberation proves that women still take the hit so that men don't have to.

Kezzia
Anger as rejection of womanhood. Her strategy = Finding the sisterhood

Nina knew that if she tried to prevent 15-year-old Kezzia from having sex with her boyfriend, or attempted to control her activities, it would backfire. As a single mum, Nina was used to shouldering the weight of seismic parenting decisions. She offered to take her daughter to the family planning clinic. Kezzia had been in the relationship for a year. I realise this sounds ridiculous to most. As adults, though, we forget how 'mature' we feel in our teens. Our minimal prefrontal cortex maturation governs our Teen difficulty with placing ourselves in a wider context. Teen Girl is a kid. But there's a vast dissonance at this point, and that's just how things have to be. Though our minds take the time they need to get there, our bodies race ahead of themselves, and any drugs we take exert their powerful effects on a body which is still trying to figure itself out. 'I just thought it can't be worse than her falling pregnant,' Nina would repeat, in anguish. She'd spent the previous few months doing her best to have conversations around consent, and had helped bring a slower pace to the progress of Kezzia's relationship. The whole family had got to know Kezzia's boyfriend well (he'd been in her class since the start of high school) and the families had become better acquainted across the year they'd been dating.

Kezzia had always been a skinny kid, but the pill

increased her appetite and, over the following six months, she gained weight. Nina took her to buy a new bikini for their holiday and found Kezzia looking at herself quizzically in the changing room mirrors.

'Do I look different?' she asked. 'My thighs ... I think they look different.'

Nina was always of the opinion that body matters should be stated frankly and honestly.

'Well, they do look a bit chunky!' she cheerily confirmed, expecting that Kezzia would agree and they could move on to a different shop.

I was obviously astounded at this retelling and Nina's nonchalance. But I knew Nina pretty well at this point. I just would have hoped that, through the course of our work, she might have retained a bit of the sensitivity and empathy I'd tried to model, and practise applying it herself. As previously discussed, it's difficult to keep how you really are *'out there'* away from the therapy room. You give yourself away in all manner of small and large ways. And Nina's abrasive and abrupt manner had been turned towards me not a few times. It was one of the reasons we'd done so much work on building her daughter's trust in Nina, and why Kezzia's shy acceptance of her mum's involvement had been meaningful.

The contraceptive pill is a life-changing resource for women. But it can also lead to a change in body shape. When you're a Teen Girl on the cusp of feeling either OK or not OK about yourself, and when you have a mum who is also – newsflash – not perfect and is trying really hard to do things better than her own messed-up experiences have left her equipped for, well, it's a lot to contend with.

Kezzia took a psychological nosedive after the bikini interaction. She had been confronted with her body being the irritating empty vessel, holding the power to suddenly, horrifyingly, house a baby – the reality of which would destroy many lives around her and would somehow be her fault if she wasn't personally taking steps to stop it – but also, somewhere around the edges of her consciousness, understanding that, if she doesn't have a baby later on, when she's meant to, many lives around her would be destroyed. Seemingly, this was the first time Kezzia arrived inside the dilemma of womanhood, perceiving her body as the pivot around which perfection needs to be defined.

When Kezzia saw her new body in the mirror, she was experimenting with being OK with it. What should Nina have said? Should she have lied and said: 'No, you look no different'? Surely we should be able to speak to our daughters in a straightforward way, so they can simply internalise this message: 'The drug I'm taking is forcing a change on my body. I'm taking it because, at this point in my life, it wouldn't work for me to have another, larger change brought onto my body.' But we know that society's strung us up so that emotions and bodies are inextricably intertwined. As women (even quite thick-skinned women like Nina), things must by default be 'our fault'. So the precipitating factor here – the 'chunky thigh' affirmation – landed agonisingly for Nina as a mother, too. Mothers and daughters are indescribably complex in their recognition and identification, but this is fundamentally also a relationship cooked up in the crucible of patriarchy.

Kezzia was angry and fell into the trap set for all women – to take it out on herself. She began to starve herself back to the weight she was. I wish I could say she's OK now, but, of course, she's not. She never will be, in one of the largest senses. Her weight's stable and her attitude towards food has moved on a bit, but, in truth, none of us recover from the moment when we realise we're screwed, however it lands for us.

What did need to get set up between all three of us – and vitally, for the longer haul, between Kezzia and Nina – was a completely transparent and frank dialogue about the most shamed parts of ourselves – our bodies – as well as the beginnings of a quite different conversation. One which gave voice to a reality that Kezzia couldn't yet begin to realise she was really angry about. Namely, the awakening recognition that society conveniently places its disgust and disdain onto women. It shovels up everything it finds messy and unwanted onto us, but simultaneously attacks us with its hateful envy of the power women hold. Because us women can apparently ruin men's lives by getting pregnant as well as cruelly hold over them this most creative trophy of all. As we know all too well, we also apparently ruin lives if we can't get pregnant. See what I mean? Teen Girl Kezzia just couldn't win. But at least knowing, in this greatest sense, that the thigh problem wasn't really about her *personally*, was a kind of triumph she could ultimately – across a lifetime – begin to build her recovery around. For Kezzia, feeling that she was part of a sisterhood that felt the same about their own entrapment in a society which slices and dices them was a kind of comfort – and allowed the beginning of a shift in perspective away from her own painfully stuck experience. For Nina, it wasn't about saying the 'one correct thing' which would help heal Kezzia. It was, instead, a paradigm shift. Conversations between mother and daughter became larger and more expansive – less about individual body parts, and more about being a woman in a strange and currently impossible world.

What we can do for Teen Girl

- Recognise our darkest feelings and try to find words for them. Even if we don't make them public.
- Help our daughters to do the same.
- Talk about bodies and the complex feelings which arise from trying to reside in them comfortably.
- Talk about the anger which arrives when we feel stared at, lusted over, dissected.
- Support Teen Girls to find ways of safely speaking out about these experiences.
- Encourage ordinary discussion around the way that we're objectified and what this means – for ourselves and in the larger patriarchal context.
- Tap down into our own memories of being a Teen Girl and be brave about confronting some of these

experiences. If we allow the memories to feel fresher, we can empathise more with those currently going through it.

- We can also use these memories to piece together why we might still have complicated feelings towards relationships, sex and our own bodies.
- When we understand where feelings have come from, and that they've been imposed on us, it can be easier to feel compassion towards ourselves. And even to find ways of moving towards healthier states of mind.
- Schools! You're getting better at teaching consent. Can we also talk about sex and bodies more openly in general, and what equality looks like? Again, talking talking talking. And listening. Properly listening. Even if we don't necessarily like what we hear.

Grab your first cheap suit! We're leaving behind the uncomfortable Teen years and diving into something far more together and glamorous ... Aren't we?

CHAPTER EIGHT

Young Woman

MANY PSYCHOANALYSTS, as well as neuroscientists, would argue that, behaviourally and at a brain developmental level, we're adolescents until we're around 30. This chapter embraces Young Woman's extended adolescence and discusses realities like entering the workplace and the role of male sexual desire as loci of potential rage. In Young Woman, we'll think about how the difference in the way we've treated boys and girls, and the divisions we instil between them, pan out as our lives hit this point. It makes for a potentially sinister read.

Based on my clinical work, I feel it's at the Young Woman stage when the patriarchy really begins to overtly *control*. At this point, even our own sense of desire is frequently siphoned and controlled through the male gaze. Female patients talk endlessly of their complicated relationship to their own bodies and sexuality, often stemming from Teen Girlhood. By opening the doors on what Young Woman discusses in her therapy, a franker conversation might become established, preventing our sex lives, as well as our professional ones, becoming further arenas of inequality and internalised frustration.

Young Woman's dating patterns come into therapy a lot. I've noticed how her tendencies, if left unquestioned, really set her up for shit relationships. Bringing her learning from childhood and what she's witnessed and been conditioned for, Young Woman struggles to be honest with men. At this life stage, we can't seem to make the connection that our angry feelings towards the terrible treatment we're getting should make us walk. Because what if *this* is our one shot at having a family? These men have us over a barrel. We put up and shut up, which sets a precedent. We *act into* outdated roles, and feel powerless to challenge them.

As Young Woman, this problem extends to our careers. Entering into the workplace when our sexual currency is at an all-time high, but our ability to confer respect is at its lowest, is a complex terrain. How do we reconcile the conundrum? We flirt, and use our bodies – because that seems to bring us power. But we feel sick about it later. You wouldn't believe – or maybe you would – the number of Promising Young Women I hear who are careful not to 'reject' affections, so as to protect their place on teams or in supervisors' favours. Even in more day-to-day experiences at work, Young Woman must pretend not to know the solution, or let someone mansplain or 'hepeat' us (a man's repetition of a woman's idea, and receiving the accolade). It feels too difficult to try to change everyone's minds about who we are and what we represent. We play the game, sell out – and, in attempting to flip the power dynamic, we're tricked into reinforcing it. I'm stunned by the repeated narratives of women patients finding themselves in 'Boys' Club' industries, from advertising to law to tech to film to recruitment to healthcare; lad-ishness, misogyny and mild to appalling levels of harassment are rife. And women repeatedly shrug it off and 'try not to let it get to me'.

Abusive relationships just love our Young Woman insecurities and people-pleasing, grateful tendencies. From careers to first, seemingly settled, relationships, this is the life stage when a particularly universal type of female anguish surfaces. As therapists, we witness a flourishing and cementing of the grim reality of earlier modelled behaviours. There is a depressing frequency of practitioners willing a Young Woman to wake up and see what a prize-winning twat he is … Often only to watch the whole car crash repeat.

What about that 'Limited' Young Man? Who is *he* learning to grow into, as he's invested with so much power and adulation? From tiny snide acorns grow oak trees of abuse. Systemically, the seeds of those gendered childhood divisions grow into the power problems of our Young Woman years. The frequency with which he got away with careless-thoughtless behaviours as a child sets us up for pain now. What begins as gameyness around 'him not deleting his dating profile' or 'leaving me on read' (when WhatsApp tells you he's read your carefully crafted message, but hasn't bothered replying) can end in domestic financial control and women contorting themselves to please, in case he calls her a nag and leaves. Welcome to our era of enlightened equality. The story hasn't changed much, as far as I hear it.

Young Women are still the ones left waiting. Young Men are still the ones who propose. Or don't. Which keeps the previous status quo ticking along nicely. And, then, there's *still* all the name-change crap if we do marry! Are you Miss or Mrs? Or are you a 'Ms', leaving everyone wondering more about your status than any other aspect of your personhood? Are you owned or does no one want you? Arguably, *what's in a name*? But it's the meaning which gets conveyed along with it, just like the colour pink. It's the energy expended, and the everyday reminder that we belong to a system in which we're *less than*. In which, historically, we belong to men.

By maximising Young Woman's sense of being defined by men in her personal and professional life, the system takes care of itself. She morphs into Adult Woman and Sandwiched Woman and Older Woman with a shit pension. It all looks extremely well organised. And it *definitely* distracts us from the knowledge of our own strength and power. In today's plutocracy, it seems, from what I see, that our impotent rage is fed by certain men feeling intimidated and pushing back against what they instinctively feel has gone too far. So a culture is assembled which works for many other men, too. Tools are employed which are known to impact a demographic who are fundamentally still oppressed. Treat 'em mean. It's always done the trick and, like kicked dogs, we come back for more … I've even seen how this works for the different treatment of sons and daughters, as they grow into adulthood. (The seeds of expectation that daughters will start stepping in as more formalised, more reliable emotional supports for parents obviously get sown years prior.) But the Young Woman years are where the physical impact begins to tell. One patient, at that point just diagnosed with ME, spoke a great deal, in fond-sounding terms, about her brother's uselessness. And, with an indulgent smile on her face, about how she 'wanted to scream!' when she was the one planning their parents' anniversary do from the waiting room of her own hospital appointment. *Very cute.*

The numbers speak for themselves. Women are still the majority victims of domestic abuse. According to 2021 World Health Organization (WHO) global preference estimates, 30 per cent of women over the age of 15 have experienced physical or sexual violence – which translates to 736 million women globally. Some sources put the figure as higher. Twenty-seven per cent of this figure describes intimate partner violence. According to the WHO, 1 in 3 pregnant women globally are victims of domestic violence. Something deep, envious and hateful can get stirred in men by pregnancy.

What I've noticed in clinic is sinister. Because, even in apparently *non-abusive* heterosexual relationships, Young Women report a disturbingly ordinary flavour of daily denigration. This spans a rainbow of behaviours, from the most subtle coercion to the cartoonishly outlandish: being shouted at, being called crazy, being called fat, leaving dirty clothes or dishes in piles for her – even just a lack of information provided about his schedule, so she's left to guess when he'll be home. Later, this evolves into poor planning around school holidays and birthdays and illnesses; Adult Woman is typically left to manage and juggle at these times. We'll revisit this happy development of low-level abuse in her chapter, but, in the meantime, let me tell you about how Young Woman Rubia saw the writing on the wall, and learnt to turn away from the 'Limited Young Men'.

Rubia
Anger as eczema. Her strategy = Ditching the terrible relationship

Rubia was suffering, as so many of us do, in the Young Woman part of her life. She'd moved through the intensely uncomfortable-in-her-own-skin phase of earlier Teen Girl years, and was now stuck in her second long-term relationship. A lot of her friends were getting engaged, and this particular guy teased her with the tantalising prospect that 'one day' he'd want to settle down. Just not yet. Rubia moulded herself around him and his apparent needs, which would eternally flex and shift. At one point, she was 'too needy'; at another, he got pissy because she arranged a trip away with friends without telling him. She just couldn't get it right. Her body was also wrong. Her friends apparently understood how to present themselves in a way which pleased him more. Whenever Rubia got a glimpse of how cruelly mediocre *he* was, she frightened herself back to him, because this was 'last chance saloon' for guaranteeing herself a family.

Eventually, I gently floated the label *sadist*. I angled the lens to show her the subtleties of the sado-masochistic system, whereby her training as an Oppressed Person in life – keeping herself in check to others' needs, prioritising their demands, fulfilling the version of her they required – came in very useful. A masochist feels pleasure at a delicately brutalising position, such as this one. Although Rubia denied that she felt pleasure at this treatment, she could see there was a certain compulsion to repeat what she'd always known. For, as we've seen, the brain is compelled to repeat – even the unhealthiest habits. Our wiring clusters into familiar, well-trodden pathways. This is how habits form – repetition across years. Unfortunately, a woman's experience is ground into our brain across all the years leading up to Young Womanhood. As Rubia found. Her body bore the hallmarks as she grappled with livid eczema. But, one day, after a night spent wondering why he hadn't returned her calls, her raw skin bleeding onto her sheets, something struck her. She rushed in to tell me the next morning: 'I don't have to do this, do I? I'm actually doing this to myself ... *He's not doing this to me ...*'

It seemed that Rubia's skin had been her red flag all along. And she finally stopped long enough to hear what it was telling her.

'I looked at my poor arms, my legs ... And I heard what you've been saying – that this relationship is a kind of self-harm. That being a masochist is a bit like scratching the eczema. I want to *so much*. I know it's bad for me, but that moment of relief, of total pleasure, it feels like it's worth it. And then, suddenly, it's not. And I feel sick with myself, and I realise what I've done. But, by then, you're trapped in the cycle. And that kind of shame – of admitting how low you've gone – keeps you going back for more.'

I agreed that, as with any kind of addiction – however the dopamine finds its release – a taste of those neurotransmitters signals to our receptors to search for more. And breaking the pattern can only really come from the person inside of the system. Rubia was ready to hear what other parts of her body were telling her. Finally, she understood what her skin – that visible site of inflammation – was telling her. Rubia, stuck in Young Woman Hell, needed to pause and listen to her symptom. Really listen. And understand that she was ready to break a cycle. Finally, she had a frank conversation with herself. Reader, she ditched him.

Frank conversations are often a problem for Young Woman. In a society which discourages the straightforward expression of their feeling, women are tainted with the reputation of bitching. From Tweenhood on, they're provided with few other outlets for aggression. Whilst Tween Boys can carry on acting like kids, Tween Girls need to find alternative spaces in which to work things through. Since the segregation persists, Young Women only have each other to help understand confusing feelings or sensations. God forbid they ask the guy who's putting them through gamey hell *what's going on with him*, or speak at a straightforward level about the pressure she feels to settle down, although she herself might be undecided, too.

With only other Young Women to share feelings with, an echo chamber – a cauldron of panic and anxiety – becomes established. Whether she's seeking a 'majority', targeted support or just some help processing feelings, the results are often the same. A lot of Young Women are left suffering when they've come away from an evening with friends, feeling like they've spoken out of turn or worried that others will ultimately find them catty or vindictive. These 'safe spaces' don't actually feel so safe – possibly because they're so intense and enmeshed. This isn't helped by social media, and the endless 'womensupportingwomen' hashtags and memes. Where are these sisters when you need something real? When you've screwed up in a human way, when your heart is cracking with your own humanity? And where are the Young Men friends who might offer a different perspective and something less merged and suffocating? *Oh yes*, as kids we were told they wouldn't be coming on the journey with us.

As it was for our younger selves, there are still few other platforms for women to express their forceful emotions, desires or aggression. So we're left with only each other as sounding boards. Close friendship groups, or other women experiencing a similar life stage or pressures, are often the only places women feel comfortable enough to air their darker or more troubling emotions around themselves in relation to others. But there are *rules* to this arrangement. When we conspire, as fellow women, to label this behaviour in a narrow and limiting way, we're ourselves exerting a patriarchal and constraining force on each other. Too often, Young Woman speaks to me about feeling 'too much' or expressing herself too aggressively or negatively in social situations. How many men, given to similar behaviours, would instead be described as 'not suffering fools' or being 'to the point' or straightforward? *Men are not bitchy*. The trouble is, when we bitch, we also run ourselves down. We attack women, we attack ourselves. We send ourselves back into powerless places, where our energy expenditure is circular and can't propel us forward.

That said, for Young Woman, there's a lot to feel bitchy

about. When I was an undergraduate, a well-known female speaker came to talk to the Young Women about our chances on graduating. Her message was: 'You can't Have It All. You have to choose.' A lot of the students left in tears. In the bar afterwards, some were inconsolable. What was the point? Had the efforts to get here been worth it? Men would never have to make the same choices. Our Young Men friends weren't invited to that undergrad speaker's event. It felt a bit like when we were split up from them at school to be told about periods. *This doesn't concern the boys – this is a female experience.* Our biology was yet again our definition. Against the backdrop of that decade of lavish opportunity that was the mid-nineties, this messaging just felt surreal. Yes, we could see that our own mums – though they'd 'gone through feminism' – were trapped between expedient career pathways, primary caring and homemaking. Looking back, it's as if our lives have been spent desperately trying to prove that speaker wrong. Yes, we've stepped up into heftier professional roles than our mums. But – as she predicted – an associated domestic revolution hasn't yet been forthcoming. And, as Adult Women, our bodies keep the score.

There's something aggressive and taunting about the reality of being told that this is what you wanted. *Enjoy it*! There's maybe even a triumphant sense from onlookers that we've woven our own nooses – how appropriately humiliating. Twenty years on from that speaker's warning, the reality (as I hear it) is that, when Young Women start having families, they enter into Adult Women reality, where part-time working actually means we cover the full five days (if not more) by working in the evenings or in the mornings by getting up before the rest of the family. We scrub ourselves out of the salary we're owed when we work on our day off because we're threatened with the notion there'll always be someone else coming up the rear. We realise that the teachings of our youth primed our care pathways for hijack, and meant we'd be the ones carrying the mental and emotional load.

Although Young Woman may arrive strident in her conviction that she'll be doing things differently, I notice, with sadness, that her behaviour in the workplace still emulates the well-behaved, nervy conditioning of her younger years. She expects senior men to address her male co-worker; she notices they talk over her in meetings or don't meet her eye. She treads on eggshells, she erases herself. She tries to pass on the manager's advice about their shared project to her male colleague. That colleague ignores her. She has a sleepless night because she'll have to face the manager. Sound familiar? But it's just not fashionable to call this out anymore, and it actually feels humiliating to admit that we're still victims of professional sexism. So we don't. But our bodies tell the story.

A three-month-pregnant patient had a doctoral interview. This was an unplanned pregnancy, whereas the professional opportunity was very much planned. She'd been working towards it for years. She made no mention to the panel of the pregnancy, but needed to run away fast in the middle of a question because the vomit had begun to force its way out (our body tells the story). The panel allowed a feedback call. They asked her, 'What happened? You were doing so well!' She couldn't tell them *now* that she was pregnant, because she hadn't mentioned it in the first place. If she tried to reapply, they might remember her. And they'd remember her as the mad one who 'forgot' to tell them she was pregnant. In truth, she knew they'd never give her the place if she declared the pregnancy. They wouldn't *obviously* be able to say that was the reason; there were a million others they could give – it was a highly competitive, funded PhD. Even if she was wrong and they wouldn't have held it against her, Young Man never has to know this dilemma. Or any kind of equivalent. True equality therefore remains a bit of an illusion.

Young Woman, pressurised to shore up her chances at having a family, sees her ambition tripped up. Even at the beginning of her career, the expected emphasis on bagging a viable partner splits her focus. So, when it comes to balancing the domestic load with her career later on, she's actually already on the back foot – unused to ever making it a full priority.

It's from this life stage that the needle on the equality scale really starts to swing away. Concealing pregnancy is one such cargo which overloads us. For our doctoral-hopeful, common sense and previous experience convinced her that bias would run against her. The onus on us as women to protect society from our inner reality is an ongoing encumbrance. What are we protecting them from? The reality that we've had sex? Or the embarrassment of brushing up against our pain if we miscarry?

It's a natural bind that women are the ones giving birth, that our bodies are the ones geared up for nourishment and provision of a baby's needs. But the trouble is, the structures underpinning all subsequent decisions assume this skew persists. So then, it does. Since a woman is often breastfeeding on maternity leave, it makes sense for her to be at home across those months. So employers make the assumption that this will be the case – and, given the choice between hiring a man who won't be feeding a baby and a Young Woman who *could* be taking that time out, they'll naturally be drawn to the man. Imagine, though, if there was a breast-pumping room in every place of employment and a fridge for milk to be stored until the end of the day! Imagine if there were creches at work. Imagine if men were offered viable paternity packages. Imagine if we were able to create more mystery around our intentions. Imagine that kind of power. It would feel a bit like … being a man.

That creep of the needle slides itself further away as Young Woman becomes Adult Woman. She won't be able to believe what lies ahead, if my patients are anything to go by. She'll have to brace herself for the fact that men still *play golf* (really!) on a weekend, or meet friends for football, or go for long bike rides, or a drink after work – frequently following being pretty absent for the rest of the week and getting home well past bath and bedtimes. She'll have to come to terms with these lonely bedtime hours as the very worst part of any day, when her own energy levels are spent and a mountain still needs to be climbed. It's not so much that men shouldn't have this opportunity to wind down in ways of their choosing, but the issue is that it's a *given*. Because they're not the ones primarily at home, the need to arrange care for children to enable them to fulfil their pastimes is simply not a requirement. Wouldn't it be better if Young Woman were told this? Could she have conversations which would protect her now, or conversations around what to do if you find you're pregnant? What are your *actual* rights in terms of employment? What can you really anticipate at work and at home by way of genuine support?

And what about the Young Woman who chooses not to have

children, or who won't be able to for physiological or financial reasons? How does society support her? How do we teach her that she has boundless value in her own right? That her life is respected for its own sake? Since we've been instructed, <u>even</u> before we were born, that we really only exist to fulfil the needs and expectations of others, this kind of messaging can quickly feel hollow and tokenistic.

My heart hurts every time I'm told by a woman that her partner's accusing her of 'nagging' when she asks him about his plans, so that *she* can plan. What a horrible, gagging word. It's sure to shut up any of us, threatened with this medieval image of a poisonous fishwife. When have you ever heard of a man being accused of nagging? The phase of life in which this crystallises is the childbearing years, even in relationships which began as partnerships, as two equally educated and enlightened people. Somehow, once children come along, all this goes out the window. We're thrown back into hackneyed old structures we're both too exhausted to battle.

As we're realising, the patterns etched into childhood steer the ways men and women are taught to interrelate. Multiple female patients have commented that having a baby is like being 'transported back to the fifties'; the potency and promises they'd experienced in their lives previously suddenly rendered apparently impossible. This is a situation which is appalling to women, once they stop thinking there's something wrong with them and confront it. My hunch is that it's also quite shocking to their partners, who were taught to dream the same dream of equality. But instead of staring down the baffling barrel of that gun and figuring out what went so wrong, it's easier to just call her a nag, or 'controlling' – words that, in themselves, are violent because they're so gagging. They cut us all off at the knees. But because that template exists already, it looks like a solution is reached. *The woman is the problem! She's expecting too much! This is on her.*

One of the core problems is that the domestic role is still so denigrated and maligned – minimised because it's invisible. Even before we have a family, the state of the home seems to fall primarily to Young Woman. Possibly because we've been inducted into the importance of keeping a nice home, and the same doesn't seem to have been expected of boys. With housework, you only know it exists when it's not done. The remorse around failing to fulfil obligations helps set women up to primarily feel guilt instead of anger. So when people then go ahead and set up in heterosexual couples, the habits are already formed. Young Woman is held accountable for living standards, by others and herself.

The other major source of repressed feeling at this, Young Woman, life stage lands with the realisation that our female bodies elicit a further differential. For this is when a lifelong, gendered interface with medical institutions really gets going, whether it's for birth control, smear tests, terminations, reproductive issues, endometriosis or yeast infections. Here we are. We've arrived. And there's no going back.

The levels of care we expect echoes the fact that, again, we're not actively on the lookout for wide-scale discrimination. We chalk up poor treatment to the general paucity of services and an overstretched, underpaid and under-respected workforce. We daren't ask for more. Or let ourselves acknowledge that women-specific provision is in a critical state.

Here in the UK, a recent chancellor reallocated a tax of a

quarter of a million, levied from tampon sales, into a pro-life organisation. The money was meant to fund charities for women. A handful of female politicians voiced their horrified objections. They were ignored. This lack of due diligence around the MO of the charities chosen is testimony to the tokenistic, scantily thought-through surface changes that have been made in our name. The offering which looks at first glance as if it helps is actually damaging us. The saccharine language which cajoles and placates diverts from the inserted dagger.

In terms of our care, the very qualities we women are known for – empathy and understanding – are used against us. We don't want to make a fuss; we don't enjoy people running around after us. It seems this has contributed to us sleepwalking into a situation in which we're collectively often treated quite badly. And we don't think to question it. Consider the enduring issues around menopause medication – shortages, reluctance to prescribe, insistence on blood testing and the paucity of training amongst GPs who are tasked with providing it. Let alone the fact that we're rarely told about the HRT passport, conferring subsidised prescriptions. Consider the hours spent waiting for a routine pregnancy review in overcrowded spaces, resembling something from a disaster movie, or the shocking treatment of women who lose babies within certain health trusts, who have to fight a court battle for their pain and loss to be taken seriously. Women can now finally request a baby loss certificate. The fact that this needs to be 'requested' at all is illustrative of the work we have to do, the interface we're forced to have with the world, when we are engaged in our most private inner grief.

It's become a very normal part of my practice to support

Young Women in getting themselves heard better within health services – beginning by listening carefully to their past experiences, which are often shocking. I wonder a lot why this doesn't get better media coverage. I can only conclude it's because women are busy, don't value themselves enough to demand better and don't have the endemic forcefulness of ego to question why this is happening to them. As well as to most other women they know.

The language of medicine evolved within the patriarchy. I'm endlessly saddened to still hear terms such as 'incompetent cervix', 'hostile uterus', 'geriatric pregnancy', 'late miscarriage' and 'adverse outcome' still borne by women as descriptions they identify with – let alone the overuse of the word 'failure' across every possible part of the fertility conversation. It's sad and further astonishing to me that we as women are left with little choice but to accept and absorb such terms being used about us, our bodies and such personally enormous experiences. Language is power, and the women I've come to know fundamentally don't feel entitled to challenge the use of such terms because they're *medical*. They've come into medical usage because, a long time ago, a man and then some other men elected to use them this way. We could talk about these painful and formative experiences in a different way now. Beginning with the fact that contemporary medical school textbooks don't even include a realistic representation of normal female genitalia, perhaps? Work is ongoing to begin this wider process of change, but it feels slow and marginalised.

It seems to me that the way we discuss our bodies (or don't) and the fact that we've learnt an inbuilt shame around so much of our biology isn't helped by our having so little ownership over the language used to describe our symptoms, and by the structures which have minimised and labelled our experiences.

In passing, during their sessions, women from this age on will frequently mention health catastrophes – that they've been suffering with a two-day migraine, or have struggled to be diagnosed with endometriosis, or have had five miscarriages in their life. Most women I see bear the scars of at least one acutely compromising health condition. Living with crippling period pains, or suffering recurrent musculoskeletal pain, or thyroid problems, or a debilitating heavy menstrual flow are seen as absolutely par for the course. These experiences are tolerated and coped with as a normal part of life. I notice that struggles around menopause and even perimenopause carry the same weary attitude – a feeling that we just need to crack on as best we can. As if our energy for believing that anyone's interested, or might be able to help, is worn thin.

I'm told again and again that successive encounters with professionals have been so dispiriting and unhelpful that women have very often given up, turned to friends for advice and tips, and, occasionally, via a form or chatroom, landed on an approach which they might at some point mention to a GP who goes beyond. But it's all the wrong way round; it's too accidental. Too few women expect to be heard, or imagine they can take up the space in a consulting room, let alone have someone think creatively in a collaborative way about options. I wouldn't blame GPs for this. GPs are my friends, allies and, increasingly frequently, patients. This is a systemic issue. It's social. This is wired in. This begins before a woman enters anyone's consulting room. It's to do with shame and being afraid to ask. It's also to do with feeling our bodies themselves are too much. The desperate experience of a cattle-like approach of queuing and overbooking for antenatal reviews, whilst elsewhere harassed midwives run between two delivery rooms, is a dismally universal theme.

It's unavoidable that women bear the load of childbearing and every aspect of pregnancy. But there's more to it than that. Take fertility, for example. Historically, the discourse around infertility and miscarriage has firmly placed accountability at the woman's door, in spite of increasing knowledge that 50 per cent of cases related to infertility are male. And that possible damaged DNA and the more general health of sperm is becoming a more widely researched area. Nonetheless, historical implication and imagination identifies the woman's body as the suspect, which, still today, often means a woman doesn't allow herself a real experience of grief if she miscarries. To miscarry is to grieve. We grieve for the loss of potential, but this gets tangled with the shame of our own *perceived sense* of incapacity. What I see is that we also feel anger – shedloads of it; particularly if our experiences are handled clumsily by family and professionals.

I frequently find myself encouraging women to connect with their feelings around miscarriage – however early a pregnancy may have been lost. It isn't possible that an experience carrying with it so much potential energy (however equivocal a woman may have felt about it at the time) fades away without a significant emotional reverberation. Energy needs to go somewhere. And if it isn't expressed, the only way is back inside.

Following the establishment of adolescence and menstruation, a woman typically only consciously confronts the realities of her female body when she becomes or looks to become pregnant. Clinically, I have all-too-extensive experience of women's psychological suffering whilst undergoing the various stages of IVF: the lack and loss of dignity, the anguish of hormonal intervention, the pain of miscarriage, the guilt felt at the financial investment – especially if these enormous efforts do not carry to term. The strain is enormous, both on a woman's mind and body, as well as on her identity and relationships.

A key problem is, again, self-blame. There's a definite sense that something going against plan in terms of fertility is the woman's fault. This doesn't exactly get challenged by the messaging of our systems around childbirth and pregnancy. Yet again, there's a sense of a woman's poor self-esteem being preyed on. Somewhere in her she might suspect this is happening, but ultimately that questioning is no match for her unrecognised rage. Her anger towards herself and others becomes inverted and internalised.

And for those whose pregnancies run to term, there's also plenty to feel enraged about. Anyone who's ever waited for routine appointments in the overstretched maternity services of the world will have experienced the familiar cocktail of irritability, dismissiveness and diminishment that are hallmarks of treatment by a staff too burnt out to be compassionate. If being pregnant and giving birth had been experiences gone through by men directly, I wonder if these services might have more importance and respect woven into them. There's a disturbing note of the factory dairy farm accompanying the treatment of these women, at possibly the most momentous and vulnerable point in their lives. Which brings me to Jasmine.

Jasmine
Anger as stomach pains and insomnia.
Her strategy = Grieving

Jasmine was someone whose body spoke volumes about her experiences. She had married as a Young Woman and was living in London with a baby daughter. Her presenting issues were insomnia and stomach pains. She'd been checked out by a GP and cleared for anything physical as the cause, and the GP had referred her for therapy to investigate what they felt may be a psychological explanation.

It took some time for Jasmine to tell me about the baby she'd lost two years previously. She'd had to give birth to him when he was full-term, having noticed that he'd stopped moving. Neither the hospital, nor her family, seemed equipped to provide her with the aftercare she required. What was striking about this was that, instead of making a complaint about the mistakes that had been made (for certainly negligence was a feature of that harrowing experience), she closed herself down: 'I don't want to sue them. Take money out of a system which is at breaking point? It's one of the reasons I lost him, I'm sure of it ...'

When family members popped over to 'see how she was', she put on a brave face: 'It wouldn't be fair to make them suffer too.' That brave face inserted itself like a mask between herself and her husband. She said she had to stop *feeling* emotionally, because if she felt anything at all, the pain would engulf her, it would eat her up. The GP put her on antidepressants, though she'd insisted she wasn't depressed. But they had nothing else to offer.

I realised that Jasmine had oceans of tears to shed, impacted inside of her. It was as if her stomach was straining under the weight of unshed tears. She was carrying them inside her like a bag of splintered glass. Her eyes were like two dry, frightened canyons staring wildly at me. What if the tears started to come? What then?

When we began to talk about her husband, Jasmine was very defensive. 'I love him to bits' (I'm always suspicious of this phrase, as it implies something destructive and fragmenting). Through gentle probing across weeks, it turned out that actually her husband was out socialising most nights after work and she hardly saw him. One day, Jasmine revealed that she was going to have trouble paying that month's invoice, because her husband had 'cut her allowance'.

'Allowance?' I asked. 'Like you'd give a child?'

'Well, like you'd give a wife,' she replied.

I didn't know where to begin with this, as Jasmine had been so conditioned by her upbringing and her husband's view of family to believe she should be grateful for his support. Even when I countered that she hadn't been able to earn money, as she was looking after their child, she said – 'Yes, this is why he pays me.' It was all just so – wrong. But it was very difficult to argue. Even now, it's hard to articulate the depth to which this feels so appallingly problematic, in a relationship and society in which we're meant to enjoy equal rights; a man meting out a meagre (and it was pretty meagre, in Jasmine's case) wage, deciding what you're worth, what your services cost. I shudder. Jasmine had no control over the family's finances, over what they spent money on together, nor over what she spent money on, as her husband expected a spreadsheet of her spending that he would approve before funding.

But apparently, he was a 'lovely man' who just happened to be very worried about money and wanted to keep a tight rein on it. He had grudgingly agreed to the therapy, since her illness was 'costing him more' through him having to take time off for childcare. It seems that, sometime after the death of her first baby, Jasmine had lost her voice. In her effort to hold back the tears, she was holding back her words too. Almost as if she was afraid that all products of her were toxic. Just as she had 'failed' to produce a healthy baby that first time, she couldn't produce healthy tears or words.

In her rage, she was punishing herself for losing her baby, as there was no one else to safely blame. As part of this punishment, she'd suggested somewhere along the way that he should pay her out of his account. Almost as if her access to it would poison their shared funds.

Through our work, I gradually helped Jasmine find her voice. But I knew that, in order to really make room for her words, we needed to let the tears flow. What were the films which always made her cry? Well, obviously, none any more. What about music? Nothing. But I kept gently insisting. Each week, I'd set homework which involved trying out different pieces of music – from classical to love songs. One day, when she was in a supermarket alone, 'Sacrifice' by Elton John piped down the sound system. Jasmine was a music snob, by her own admission. One of the reasons the crying exercise was so difficult for her was because she approached it so intellectually. But, on this day, something about the conflation of the weather – a light spring drizzle – and maybe some visual cue from the pet aisle she'd walked past, and she was transported back viscerally and suddenly to the death of her cat, her first beloved pet. The tears came. The tears of her child self; abandoned, without inhibition, anguished and magnificent. Jasmine ran out of the supermarket and into a neighbouring alley and let them flow. They came from the pit of her stomach; they came from her guts. They came from her deepest, flayed internal organs. Poor Jasmine, she howled. Poor Me. Poor Baby Boy. Poor Us. Poor Daughter who would never know an older brother. Poor Husband, chased into a mean and partial part of himself, pushed away by the unspoken, unexpressed pain between them. What a gulf this had been. And here was her voice. The words she'd been afraid to give herself flowed out of her with her tears. They didn't cut her insides, as she feared they would. They washed them, they soothed them. 'Hydrotherapy' we called this together. She said that she'd read somewhere that people with ulcers with no access to other treatments benefited from drinking lots of water. She felt this was what she was giving herself. The raging fire which had burnt her inflamed stomach so painfully was now quenched by her own tears.

She's now learnt to use this voice in her marriage. Having *my* voice as backing gave her the initial courage to do so, but then she found her footing and there was no stopping her. The two of them began to speak. Jasmine used the words – and the tears – which our work had enabled her access to. Her husband began his own therapy, which meant that the conversation between the two of them gained in confidence and risks were taken. They exposed their emotions to each other again. And the equity rebuilt – emotionally and financially.

A note around money for the Young Woman: get this sorted. I find myself struck – again – by an atmosphere of the fifties, as women describe to me that the husband manages all the money and accounts and that she 'doesn't really know what's going on'. What is happening here?! According to the Duluth 'Power and Control Wheel', which denotes categories of financial abuse, giving someone an allowance/not allowing access to family income registers high as a predictor of power imbalance. And likely suggests that more is going on under the surface and at probably unaddressed levels, which adds up to women being in weaker positions. This is certainly borne out by evidence I hear in the room. It's also equally alarming to hear how many women seem satisfied or even 'suggest' that this is how money is shared. Let's get serious about equality and erosion of power, please!

Jasmine's story highlights another distressing reality: the

way in which mothers of babies who are stillborn are treated. There's been some very recent progress made in how women who miscarry are cared for (women picking embryos out of the bins they were told to throw them into or scrabbling around in hospital toilets trying to salvage tissue for testing are just a couple of traumatic experiences women recount). But, as yet, the experience of women delivering stillborn babies doesn't seem to have come under as much scrutiny. The fact that women are expected to deliver stillborn babies naturally, and receive little understanding about the ongoing support they'll need, is highly concerning. A coffin labelled 'hospital babies', positioned in a chapel and surrounded by several mourning families, seems to be the norm. Those of my patients who have experienced a stillbirth still, at some deep level, blame themselves for the baby's death. It doesn't seem possible for their minds to quell questions about their ultimate accountability. They're eternally flung back on the memories from a distorted position of responsibility; I should have done more, what if I'd sought help sooner? Although post-mortems and medical professionals attempt to disabuse her, forcing her to deliver the baby naturally seems to her a grotesque punishment and enduring psychological scar, which communicates the opposite.

The women I've worked with whose babies have died whilst still inside of them report to me feeling like meat, like 'livestock', as if they're simply a uterus containing something appalling. By implication, they're made to feel they've done something wrong and bad, and that they carry a sickness which must be shut away and not spoken of. They deliver their dead babies in crumbling wards, to the sound of live babies crying in neighouring bays. Though there are offers of counselling, if 'she would like', a counsellor needs to come in and take the hand of this woman – she doesn't have the means to get herself into *their* room.

This is happening at many major teaching hospitals. Women who thought they had a say in their lives find themselves the only woman in the room when the needle is brought in to stop the baby's heart or being told to buy a doll's dress for the baby's cremation since none of the 'real' clothes fit. Later, she will gaze in mute horror at a coffin loaded up with stillborn babies; her own abdomen still distended from carrying one of them.

The Royal College of Obstetricians and Gynaecologists discusses the importance of giving birth naturally to a dead baby for the woman's physical health, and for the health of future births. But, time and again, it occurs to me that the psychological impact is seemingly underconsidered, which doesn't get addressed, because how would a woman be able to leave 'feedback'? So they eventually come and tell me. I'm horrified. Every time. But my focus needs to be on helping this woman *now*. And so her immediate raw screams of pain echo through empty hospital corridors, shouting into the wind. Nothing changes.

Young Woman begins to understand, even if only in her unconscious, that the field of medicine, populated almost exclusively by men until the twenty-first century, has left an unquestioned legacy in its wake concerning the female experience; their needs, their mental health. The inescapable facts of biology – we carry the baby, we give birth to the baby, our body continues to sustain the baby – creates a foundation for dismissal and blame. Ownership of the terrain on which infants are created spells our accountability. At an intellectual level, we understand that the work of bringing babies into the world is best viewed as a shared task. Practical realities challenge this. All too easily, woman becomes her womb, paperwork, and not much more.

Young Woman discovers that this attitude pervades all aspects of female care. It's a sorry reality that abortion still needs a two-doctor sign-off in the UK, creating untold anguish and unnecessary emotional suffering. This technicality overwrites the 1861 legislation that termination of pregnancy remains a crime in Great Britain under the Offences Against the Person Act. That this legal quirk continues to hold sway indicates the extent to which women are still not convincing custodians of their own bodies. Essentially, there's a criminal underpinning to the decision to have an abortion in the UK. Campaigners and certain politicians are working hard to give women rightful control over their own bodies. The reality these lobbyists face is that those they approach for support don't actually realise the status of abortion here. In my therapy practice, I keenly felt the overturning of Row versus Wade in the US, and the ripple effect on the psyches of women everywhere. How can we, as Western democracies, begin to challenge Afghanistan, Iran, India on their treatment of women, as we witness the most basic body rights of women burn on our own watch?

Over here, women's health is under-researched and under-resourced. Women from Young Womanhood onwards approach me to speak about the debilitating effects of conditions as far-reaching as migraine, premenstrual syndrome (PMS), endometriosis and perimenopause, and extending to vaginal dryness, or vaginismus, or laxity post-birth. One woman waited four years to have painful scar tissue removed following vaginal tearing. She wasn't able to have the second baby she'd planned because she couldn't have sex without vomiting in pain.

These women turn to me, their *psychological* therapist, for support – very often because they haven't received any other kind for the devastating impact of these health disorders. From where I'm sitting, it no longer feels possible or ethical to ignore the number of women wondering aloud whether they'd have been treated so dismissively if they'd been male. An increasing number of women now take their male partners into appointments with them, reporting that they feel they have more of a chance of being heard and taken seriously by doing so.

The majority of women I've spoken with on the topic of childbirth, in my professional and personal life, are in some way traumatised by their experiences. What I'm left wondering is, is this normal? Should having babies feel so harrowing, or are we doing it badly? Patients tell me that addressing the over-medicalisation and patriarchal control of childbirth can be very helpful. Midwife-led or homecare certainly seem to provide more natural-seeming solutions. But, in reality, understaffing can make these options dangerous and create trauma around unplanned intervention. I worry that, again, tokenistic provision of birthing centres, if they can't be safely staffed, leaves women feeling less in control and more exposed to danger. Dehumanised.

The dearth of financial support and academic research into issues affecting women, from childbirth to menopause to fibromyalgia, betrays the classically dismal view of services which would benefit women's health and actually help them contribute revenue. Horrifying findings in the media bear out the tendency towards ignoring what women are telling professionals about their own bodies. The drift of non-clinically-trained hospital managers towards budgets and policy overwrites the teaching 'listen to the patient'.

You can see how disruptive it is to steer women towards their anger – to encourage them to understand their rage, to understand that they don't need to put up with dismissive treatment – in order to gently free them from assumptions and low expectations which are outmoded, but still seem to linger unchallenged. And to provide them with more of a sense of control and a stake in the structures which are allegedly there to support them. Professionals and services need to partner up with women and move forward together as a team around the woman's body. They need to think across the longer term, in order to support women's faster physiological and psychological well-being. Because, ultimately, if we're only being cynical and capitalistic, society would have a larger, stronger workforce.

As things stand, my female patients are inclined to conserve the little energy they have when they're sick. Expecting insufficiency from their physical healthcare provision con-tributes to less suffering in the here and now. We bottle it up instead – pain on top of pain. It's difficult to build confidence in the way we talk about our bodies and the needs of our bodies when we learn from a young age that these attempts could fall very flat. Because our elders internalise and hand down these dismal expectations, we mirror this. Patients describe finding themselves apologising for taking themselves to medical appointments, just as they apologise for their therapy sessions. Confusion and anger about what we're entitled to are the hallmarks of growing up in a society hardwired to diminish our experience and our pain. We desperately need to do better as professionals. And, as women, we need to take ourselves by the hand and lead ourselves firmly into that room. *Expect* that professional to work with you as an equal, rather than being patronising and diminishing.

As I listen to the countless body-bound horror shows of Young Woman, from medical termination to sexual assault to stillbirth to periods so painful you pass out, I'm struck by the reality that our biology is in many ways still our destiny. I despair that this needs to be the case; that we somehow haven't evolved past the point where having an open space inside of us forever renders us vulnerable, like a sort of treacherous sinkhole. But isn't the real issue that 'I'm fine'? The coping *despite*? We do have these body parts. They do need our (and *your*) care. Can we just talk about this, please?

Our enforced muteness seems to apply to any negative experience involving our reproductive organs. Heaven help the Young Woman attempting to pursue a claim of sexual assault. From where I sit, this looks bleak. As part of the legal process, doubt will be poured onto her account. As if this double violation is not harrowing enough, her own vulnerability is used against her. That which made her at risk of attack in the first place is used against her in judgement. Having a vagina, the body part she's attacked for, is also what makes her weak in court. A process presided over and legislated by men can never hope to provide the neutrality and safety required by a woman publicly exposing herself through trial. Society has cleverly structured our brains, through its careful conditioning from babyhood, to self-blame. We doubt ourselves. We feel weak and *unbelievable*. That literal space within us, our uterus, makes us more susceptible to being filled up; in this case, by other people's narratives. The female patients I've seen through sexual assault cases are all made to feel as if they did something wrong – both at the time of attack and by the scrutiny of others afterwards. Kellice was the perfect illustration of how our own minds seek to protect us by throwing us under a kind of horrendous, self-annihilating bus.

Kellice
Anger as post-traumatic stress disorder (PTSD).
Her strategy = Tackle the rage head-on

In order to fully protect identities, Kellice is actually several patients over the years aggregated into one, because these experiences in young women's lives are horrifyingly common. Kellice was a victim of sexual assault whilst I was working with her. Kellice, unlike others, decided to report the case, and I did my best to support her through it. I had to provide evidence, which is never helpful, because, as previously mentioned, you can only couch the narrative in terms of 'what the patient has told me', which immediately makes the patient feel that, somehow, I'm not on their team in the way they'd previously believed.

When I recall 'Kellice' (i.e. more young women than I can bear to count) and what happened to her, I feel sick. Not just because of the hell she was forced to endure, but because of the repetition of the attack at the hands of our policing and legal system subsequently, as she sought justice. I feel it deep in my stomach. Disgust. Rage. That, knowing what I know about what these young women tell me, all I can offer up are my paltry, beige notes or an unfeasible letter. It disgusts me. It shames me. Is this all any of us can do for each other, whilst she feels naked, stripped and humiliated to her bones in front of parents, cross-examiners, a system geared *against* her? How can we still be so unevolved and barbaric? How can women's bodies and experiences still be treated so disdainfully? It's as if we're dragged through the dirt at the back of a wagon, braying crowds and faceless executioners looking on. I've seen it all the way through – from her life before an attack, to the attack itself, to this shameful embarrassment of a judicial experience, women are shredded and spat out the other side. And it ruins them.

Kellice started to suffer with terrible PTSD symptoms following the attack. These worsened as she was forced to relive the experience at the hands of the police and during the trial. We found that treating the rage behind, and as a result of, the memories helped to alleviate some of these (themselves traumatising) symptoms as they arose. As her intrusive thoughts surfaced, we envisaged sawing them up with vicious power tools. Kellice felt the need to match the violence she had experienced with her own means of expression. She would draw men and cut their heads off, make effigies out of pillow towers and mash them up with her body, stab wooden spoons repeatedly into piles of coats. She had to resist inverting the feelings and re-experiencing them as attack. She had to aggress them out of her. More work for her but better this way than any of her previously life-changing symptoms.

The entire experience of working this closely with women's psyches, and the emotional fall-out of sexual violence, underscores to me the medieval limitations of the legal system, of how ill-equipped we are to protect women and to ensuring their fair treatment – and how the symptoms women are left with as a result of their experiences feel like a double attack. These cases live on always in my core, where they'll eat me up until something real changes.

What we can do for Young Woman

- Men need to ask.
- We need to tell. *Not ask*. Tell.
- Say 'vagina' at least 16 times a day. We need to address this body shame. Now. We're all upholding it.
- It's also cultural to some degree. Would it help if, as in Scandinavia, we all start doing some naked sauna time?
- Say it. Say it all. Especially when you feel the pressure to shut it down.
- Imagine looking your male co-worker/boss in the eye and saying one of your 16 'vaginas' to him. That locus of eternal shame and vulnerability can finally become a source of audacious mental power.
- Tell people what you need.
- Support other women – at work, college and in families – to be open and honest about our bodies collectively. 'Do you mean your vagina?' for example.
- Support other women as a first reflex. That instinct is data-backed.

- Stand up tall and get back in the room. Vagina first.
- If you're planning a family, talk this through properly. Will he take parental leave? Will he get up when the baby wakes in the night? Will he take time off when the kids are sick? Is this going to look like Team Together, or a solo show?
- Employers! Bring in some HR training right now around men respecting women and understanding boundaries and power abuse. Are they really listening to Young Woman? Do they know how?

Buckle up and grab your oxtail soup. You're going to need muscle for the next haul. Adult Woman: the apex of patriarchal power play, the prime point for pill-popping.

CHAPTER NINE

Adult Woman

ADULT WOMAN HAS navigated those earliest employment years, has all the young kids (if she's going to have them) and, from what I see, frequently doesn't have dynamic parents she can turn to for help. They may be off living their happy retirement. Many certainly seem very busy. Or are located far away because trying to Have It All meant that Adult Woman might live in a city she didn't grow up in. She may even have had to move for her partner's work or perhaps those parents might now be a bit too old to help. Whatever the reason, Adult Woman does without. Though she may be smarting from the rejection of this, she finds clothes which fit her unrecognisable body, and ploughs on.

If this is the time point in which she's having her first baby, Adult Woman has a lot of other exciting things to look forward to. From navigating a health system stacked against her to returning to her career 'proper' after maternity leave, sleep-deprived and glued together with milky vomit and nappy cream, yes, indeed, Adult Woman is where I see female rage at arguably its supercharged, its most visceral – and at its most sublimated and physicalised.

Hitting the glass ceilings, crashing headlong into absurd inequality and tasting the futility of a circular system are de rigueur across the Reproductive Years – mirroring the extent to which our hands are tied to do much about it. Typically, we bury the rage deep inside and watch it emerge as a host of different symptoms. In this chapter, we meet a range of women, diminished and denigrated in various ordinary ways, and consider how we can reclaim our right to feel furious about this total BS. The psychological navigation of *not* having children also features here. In recognising the absurdity of society's attempts to regulate us, we can crack on with demanding better.

Whilst it's undeniable that women's neurology changes on childbirth, I believe that patriarchal structures exploit those biological events. A patient of mine suffering with a feverish virus asked her male partner to pop to the mini supermarket and pick up apples, as their little girl needed fruit for her packed lunch. The dad came back with a mango and, when questioned, huffily retorted that he wouldn't be going back out. It was so deliberately and aggressively off the mark in terms of what could easily be accommodated in a lunchbox, showing a total lack of connection with domestic duties. But it was also a clear act of aggression towards his ill wife and his daughter: 'You won't bother asking me to do that again!'

As soon as we have to ask for things – 'Would you mind collecting/making lunch/completing this form/taking X to this appointment?' – we're aware of daring to place the burden on that other person. We also reinforce our and everyone else's assumption that this stuff is indeed our burden. This is The Load – the thinking, the shouldering of emotions, the decision-making. And, as we've seen, we've been primed to carry it since before we were born.

The paradox is that this invisible work, for all time tied to the role of homemaker/mother, and for all time running alongside any other profession, is as equally denigrated as it is *allegedly* venerated, leaving a woman to question what value she has if she isn't also bringing in an income. A frightening number of women come to me telling me that their professions have had to go as a result of the demands of mothering. The 'lie' they were sold about being able to Have It All just hasn't materialised. They've *really* tried but it seems the stitch-up is complete when we consider just how much mothers are blamed for any perceived imperfection in family life.

In psychology, we're taught to view problems through the lens of the biopsychosocial. That is, as a complex enmeshment and interplay between these key factors. How, then, have certain conditions become so divorced from being viewed through this prism? How have they been reduced down to something purely physical, which can be labelled as a catch-all and treated with medication?

Postnatal depression is a good example of this. I've treated a number of Adult Women who've been diagnosed, either professionally or by worried family members – or even by themselves – with PND. The mystery to me at this point is that we view this feeling state as a separate, discrete subtype of depression. From my professional viewpoint, who *wouldn't* feel absolutely mown down and crushed by this vast transformation in one's life? Yes, of course significant hormonal changes are at play. But, as with PMS, if we put all of a woman's problems down to this, it allows us to locate the issue in *her* and *her messed-up chemistry*, rather than looking at the wider picture. Which, for men, may mean that more ownership for this shared state needs to be accepted.

Whilst this isn't a denial of the PND diagnosis, which is a potentially dangerous one, it *is* a plea to have a different kind of conversation around it. Let me try to articulate the key issues at play for new mothers with previously no formalised experience of depression: you're never alone; you're so sleep-deprived you may have begun to hallucinate; and you're responsible for the care of a tiny, entirely dependent, vulnerable human 24 hours a day. Never again will you tear from home with keys and a mobile. Instead, you'll have just about scraped together a wagonload of nappies, spare clothes, bottles, dummies and blankets, only to have the baby wake and begin screaming for a feed, or do a violent liquid poo that soaks through all clothing and bedding and requires immediate changing. And remember, the baby can't help you to get their clothes on. They can't roll to the side or put their arm in a sleeve. Every effort needed by you is so tiny and fiddly and slow. If you live in an apartment, up you go again. Do you lug the buggy with you? Is it safe to leave it all in the hallway? Can you change the baby on the communal floor?

In an alternative scenario, baby has finally decided to nap at 11am, following a night where the most consecutive sleep you achieved was 40 minutes. Wrestling out of your milk-/vomit-sodden nightshirt, you head for the shower. Baby wakes up when you've been in it for three minutes and are just beginning to enjoy the warming comfort of the jet. Agonised, you tear away from the soothing water, feeling the icy fingers of the hallway land on your dripping skin. Do you bring baby back into the bathroom and try to find something soft to lay them on or ditch the shower entirely, having washed little more than the back of your head? Your hair dangles in cold, tangled tails down your freezing back, but your breasts start to shoot out milk, and the baby's anguished face says it all.

You're angry and choked in ways that you could never have imagined. Your husband intimates or even states outright that his friends' wives are finding this so much easier. He's out socialising after work until midnight and wonders why you feel *your* life is forever changed, why you're asking yourself, What have I done? And don't get me started on the number of male partners who dare to allege that their newly extended working hours are 'So I can support *you*!' What about the fact that your wife/girlfriend has put her career on hold so that *you* can have a family? What about that? The danger with terming feelings of impotent rage around new motherhood 'postnatal depression' is that it lets off the hook those around you – the people who apparently were so thrilled about you providing them with a son/daughter/niece/nephew/grandson/grandchild.

Wider society can also avoid addressing its pretty paltry support system. I'm not even talking about the facilities, I'm talking about the discussion around childbirth, which is normalised as 'baby joy' and 'blessings' and 'gratitude' and fails to take into account the lived, shredded-up reality. You've been literally forced inside out and you're afraid to go for a poo in case everything rips open again and you bleed out into the loo. The brain registering the near-death experience of childbirth as trauma is entirely plausible. Up to 45 per cent of women experience it that way; waking up sweating in the night, flashbacks, panic attacks. It's all up for grabs.

I hear about how family and friends are keen to be present for cuddles and photo opportunities, but often don't think or don't have time to offer something more substantial, which might promote your human need for care or your sense of self. Or help ease your chronic RSI from lifting baby, or your sleep deprivation, or let you use the loo alone. Family members often step away from further responsibility for the well-being of this entity which they were so keen you bring into the world. They might have even pressured you to go ahead and get pregnant. They might actually be too old to really be able to help much in practical terms. And your female friends are busy trying not to crack inside of their own lives. The lack of recognition may not be deliberate, but with little apparent acknowledgement of your conflicted feelings, Adult Woman can only conclude 'the problem must lie with me'.

If other people aren't offering to hold your baby so that you can eat or sleep or have a shower, it must mean that having a newborn is a breeze. And if you're struggling, then *you* must ergo be the problem. If you're tearful, agonised or even questioning your decision, then you must have *postnatal depression*. If you're failing to adopt a bovine pose of beneficence and benign serenity, all decked out in White Company gear, then something is pathologically wrong. Since we as women are not permitted rageful feelings around birth and bearing infants, if we're struggling with any of it, the risk is we'll be branded with a convincingly harrowing diagnosis, which robs us of our individual and important responses – and everybody else of any responsibility.

I have a sense from where I sit that this tendency is growing. The apparently 'skewed' numbers during the pandemic, where new mums were reported twice as likely to suffer, were revealing and truthful. I worked remotely through that whole first lockdown, barely leaving my room for air, back-to-back with frightening situations of domestic abuse and attempted suicide. The patients I feared for most were the new mums and their babies. They were in real danger. Which says everything about the vast levels of support needed around a mother and a baby – literally, a village. How many modern Adult Women can boast a village?

The more Adult Woman is instructed to expect from her life as a whole, as well as her experience of parenting, the more susceptible she is to feelings of wrongness or negativity around the reality of the experience. What feels baffling to me is that women's lives were meant to expand to fit a family and a great job. But where are the men in this? We know what it takes to raise a baby. So, from a logistical point of view, how is it possible for that same person to still do that *and* have a glittery career? She's highly educated, she's immensely capable, but feminism didn't grow her another pair of hands.

What my female patient now sees, when she becomes Mother, is that she quickly risks losing her hard-won stake in society. She's patronised by health visitors, who see a baby hitting its milestones and being well cared for. Her frozen, baffled gaze is ignored. How did this assumption come to pass, that *she's* left holding the baby, whilst her partner – her previous *equal* – resumes life as normal? Adult Woman possibly doesn't have the language to articulate this. It feels absolutely the last taboo. And no one wants to hear it, because she's so lucky to have been blessed with a baby. Especially at her age!

WOMEN ARE <u>ANGRY</u>

For many Adult Women, maternity leave means taking a financial hit. Even more so for those who decide to take a career break at this point to prioritise family, or perhaps change professions. These women patients report a huge feeling of discomfort at no longer holding a financial stake, at being placed in a position which means they have to ask for money or are given an allowance by their husbands (allowances, to remind you, are legally classed as abusive). When men wince (yes, *really*) at their partner asking for extra money for maternity or baby clothing, she feels both angry but also cowed. Again, we have women being *forced to ask*. I remind her of the optics of this, that this is a form of financial abuse. But the damage to her self-respect, and the relationship, has been done.

What I've seen in clinic is that gay couples clearly suffer twice in this respect – in a society geared towards the model where at least if Adult Woman is hitched to the wagon of a better paid man, she stands to receive a bit of protection. In a same-sex female partnership with children, the maternity hit arrives, but the partner who continues to work will also, over her lifetime, expect to be earning less than men. This can bring pressures and tensions into a relationship which I feel are really The Voice of Patriarchy, more than anything to do specifically with the couple themselves. If one woman spends a lifetime losing out, two women lose out in ways which are difficult to properly quantify.

With many women waiting until their thirties before having their first baby (cruising for that *geriatric pregnancy* …), it could be argued that she *is* lucky – and pitted against the pain of childlessness when a baby is so desperately desired, these complex postpartum feelings can seem at best spoilt and at worst heinous.

This seems to further shut her down. And, by now, we know what happens to internalised rage ... She's *wrong* to be feeling this way, when she knows women – friends, family members, colleagues – who would be desperate to have a chance at this version of life. And because we allegedly have so much mastery over our bodies and fertility now, she can't argue that this baby was a surprise. So it seems outrageous to others when conflicting feelings arrive with said baby. This lack of understanding from those around her contributes to the frequently cheated, enraged and ashamed feelings she tells me about. Essentially, we aren't allowed to have two experiences at once.

Adult Women patients wonder how, when they're so used to being treated as equals in the world of work, study and partnership, it's possible to be so demoted into this valueless role. The man's important stresses at work are still king. These are *real*. He can't really be expected to take the baby when he gets home. He *has* to give the baby back. Sorry lady – but the work which brings home the bacon obviously trumps this soft version of labour and load. These micro moments of maternity leave shape the future of things to come.

My Adult Woman patient is humiliated by her biology, by the leakiness and softness and fragility of her position – both in societal terms and in her sense of stability and standing within her relationship. And now everyone has an opinion. They may not have had a clue about what she did professionally, and had to butt out there. But they have a lot of great ideas about how to get babies fed and sleeping and able to 'self-soothe' and how much fresh air they need. *Shut up new mum*! You're a beginner again. Having headed up a department professionally, you're now completely clueless. Your stock is low, your self-esteem is lower and you're extremely angry about this denigration and demotion. But you're not allowed to say so, because *you really wanted this.*

From my therapist's chair, I'm privileged to see how this dynamic plays out for Adult Woman, once children are older: the new exasperation which arrives once school adjusts into its habit of phoning *you* if there's a problem, or the reality of struggling through the day after a night nursing a sick child, downing caffeine and ibuprofen through meetings, having hurriedly organised an agency sitter to look after them. We don't doubt what our colleagues feel when we have to run back home for vomiting, or a fall from a climbing frame, or nits (yes, really). The woman. The mum.

And that's an exceptional day. What about the ordinary days, when assumptions land on us to hold The Load in mind – the drop-offs, the pick-ups, the nanny interviews, the nursery visits, parents' evenings, toenail cutting, dental appointments, the meal planning – *another* meal? Already? The homework, the uniforms … It's a job. And it's not a job plus a job. It's a job *multiplied* by a job. At no point did anyone warn us we'd be doing two full-time jobs. That detail was left out, amid a blur of false assurances about how family members would help, and employers would make allowances, and friends would be supportive. Having It All actually means *doing* it all. And it serves men and patriarchal structures to pretend they'll offer their understanding hand before it's too late, and we realise that was a lot of convincing hot air.

This abandonment is echoed across the experiences of women around the bodily process of creating families. Many male partners seem highly resistant to revisiting a woman's feelings around birth trauma and postnatal agony of any kind. It might take years before a woman is ready to revisit and process this time. In my experience, men push back on engaging here, almost as if they feel accused in some way. Maybe they prefer to avoid it for fear of reinciting their own anxiety. But it's a privilege to have that choice. A privilege which backfires. Because it's her gagged rage which I see in my consulting room. And I don't dare call it *anything else.* Least of all PND. The agonising emotional experience of working with women such as Tamara has taught me better.

Tamara
Anger as locked-in despair. Her strategy = Friendship and community

Tamara was receiving care by a specialist community perinatal mental health team. Her enduring symptoms were feelings of hopelessness, of shutdown, of dread, and she'd been formally diagnosed with **PND**. Tamara was brittle and organised and had all the latest *things you need*. Apparently, their apartment was so packed full of baby gadgets, there was actually no room to walk safely through it, which added to her intrusive predictions of falling with or onto the baby and harming him.

Tamara hadn't realised that she was furious. Her family had been so desperate that she have a baby. And where were they now? Her parents lived outside the UK and, once they'd stayed for the first week, that was all the support she was clearly going to get from them. Her friends were dispersed – no one lived locally, nor were they around during the day – and her husband just didn't seem prepared to make any kind of allowance. Her work colleagues had all sent flowers and cards and more baby stuff and it was as if this was an adequate substitute for any other kind of physical presence or support.

What Tamara needed was for someone to listen and understand what she was actually feeling, rather than giving her a shiny new piece of equipment or telling her she had something wrong with her. Motherhood is a lonely business; we're not really wired for doing it in this isolated, individualistic way.

She was sent to a bleak-sounding 'support' group for new mothers. Tamara felt confounded and misunderstood there. 'They made us look as if we were ill. But we weren't ill. People just didn't understand what we were feeling. And we felt too ashamed to articulate our feelings, so we let them call us ill.' She later cried to me, 'How can we still be in this position? It feels Victorian! I'm being rebranded a Hysteric! I'm not depressed! I'm fucking furious!' But it seemed the more Tamara expressed anything, the more fearful those around her became and the more the bars of 'care' around her tightened.

Tamara came to see me on the recommendation by someone she'd met at the group. At the point we began work, Tamara was quietly livid. Initially she was spiky, and afraid to show me her emotion, because she thought she'd get herself into further 'trouble'. That she might end up in hotter, scarier water by revealing the depths of her feeling to me; that, somehow, I'd be obliged to feed this back to the care team. Tamara hesitated to commit to the work.

She kept saying, 'Something's wrong, something's wrong.' Over time, I began to help her believe *her* version of events – that it was the world around her that had got it so terribly wrong. Why wouldn't she feel betrayed and furious? This was not the promise she'd been sold. Added to the new and overwhelming psychological position she'd found herself in, for which she'd been completely unprepared, having experienced no obvious discrimination in her life to date, was the physical trauma she'd incurred during the birth.

Having given birth to her son vaginally (again, she felt she'd been mis-sold a fantasy about what this would involve) and come away with third-degree tearing, she was flayed physically too. Four months on from the birth, she still felt afraid to do a poo in case she tore the repaired tissue. 'This is not my body! This is not my life!' I should add that she was caring for the baby well physically, and no one had concerns about her capacity here, but both family and professionals did keep addressing her as if she was disabled, and this simply did not fit with her reality.

She had tried to join the local NCT new baby class, but had found people competitive and pushy. 'No one listens to each other – it's just about who's doing what the best, whose baby is the most advanced, and who has the best stuff ...' It struck me how similar this experience of new motherhood is to the experience of Tween and Teen Girls, and I shuddered to realise how so little changes – how so much of our lives as women is pitted *against* rather than *towards* each other.

Just as Billie, who we met in Chapter Six, had, Tamara badly needed a friend. She needed to feel the support of other women. When we team up with others going through something similar, that sense of meaning and connectedness we're longing for can begin to seed. Tamara's experience of being so in her own head with her feelings infinitely worsened her symptoms. On my veiled encouragement, and at her reluctance, Tamara started going to a baby swim class. We talked through her feelings about the changing rooms – hair, plasters, overflowing nappy bins, and so on. We reflected on her rage about each of these aspects – why is it so difficult to keep things in better order? – and we explored her feelings of trepidation when she started chatting to a particular mum each week, who asked her to come for a coffee after the third class. Why did this feel so difficult? Essentially, people had badly let Tamara down. She'd been left literally holding the baby. Why would she want to allow someone else to do the same thing?

However, by identifying the obstacle to letting some-one get close to her, Tamara cautiously began to trust this new woman in her life. Her anger needed a friend to couple up with. And, in Fatima, she found one. Though they came from very different backgrounds, they had something huge in common – their sense of being let down and abandoned, and how furious they felt about it. Their babies grew, and so did their confidence. Tamara took to Fatima the insistence I laid on this being a vast moment in their lives; that nothing would ever be the same again – not on a physical, nor at an emotional level – and that they were allowed to have strong feelings about that. They began to gather more women around them and, within the space of a few months, had begun to call themselves The Life Raft. They became happier and more joyful, and would go for day trips and later camping trips with the dads. Their louder, more expectant shared voice seemed to translate back into the home, and the men began to listen, respect and respond to what was being asked of them. They were being asked to step up and share The Load. And they gradually accepted.

When a woman arrives in my consulting room with a diagnosis of PND, she will often eventually articulate that she doesn't know where her old life went. I'm *not* saying that PND is the label society wrongly gives women who struggle with these realities. I *am* asking for a more fruitful, productive conversation about how we label mothers who are in psychological pain.

Maternity pay from Adult Woman's employer dramatically reduces at around six months, after which time she can suddenly find herself dependent on her husband. Instead of assuring women that it's OK, he's planned for this, her partner's panic at carrying the financial load can be expressed as aggression. Women from diverse economic backgrounds tell me that their husbands jab at them for having spent money on an item of clothing needed for their changing bodies, a small piece of furniture or something for the baby … 'ours' suddenly becomes 'mine'; '*My* money is being spent.' When the woman points out that the specifics of the situation aren't of her choosing or that she could return the item, the man is contrite. But a fortnight later, she has to ask again.

What I'm saying is – women feel diminished, frightened, powerless, trapped. But this behaviour seems to work regardless of industry or wealth. This problem is systemic, it's rooted back in Girl Baby – we saw certainly how in Young Woman the early training opened the floodgates for this. And the same system is still keeping Adult Woman in a very restricted place: anxious, without capacity and with the fast feeling that all of her previous self-worth is dissolved. The solution? Go back to work. The problem with this? All of the domestic habits that have been established across this time remain. It's just that, now, she has to factor in childcare (a job in itself) and the professional juggle alongside.

This means that, when she returns to work, she's typically doing so from a position where she feels she's lived a day already. In my experience, men frequently leave the house early to go to the gym, or for a meeting, or just to get ahead of a busy day, with very little need to consider the constraints of the domestic, and what planning may be required within the household that day – from PE kits to packed lunches to someone being taken sick in the night and requiring a day off school. If a marriage or partnership ultimately breaks down (which we know the poor division of The Load contributes to), watch how many husbands change their childcare days and stretch the arrangement and gaslight around custody agreements to suit themselves – even schedules which have been drawn up in the courts. You'll all have heard versions of it. You may indeed be living through it. Women are punished both outside and inside the institution of marriage.

When inside of the institution which is meant to protect her so well, the expectation that women will arrange gifts and remember her partner's family birthdays also seems normalised. And she's frequently conferred responsibility for logistical planning wherever humans are concerned, which seems to kick off as soon as couples even just cohabit. Remember the domestic expectations weaving their wiring into Young Woman's life? Well, Adult Woman sees those evolve and hard-bake. Our conditioning creates the landscape for ever more extreme exploitation. This goes for emotional exploitation too. One patient told me with incredulity that her male partner had asked why the stress he was expressing landed so hard in her. 'I don't get overwhelmed when you tell me about your feelings!' he argued. She tried to explain that a lifetime of conditioning, of leaping to take responsibility for the feelings of a room, meant that others' emotions really do have to resonate more for women. He didn't understand what she meant.

Another Adult Woman patient described her disastrous journey home from a family holiday ... They should have been back in London by lunchtime. They were back at midnight, having spent seven hours in a European departure lounge. Her tiny children were surprisingly unruffled by the experience – mostly because their mum was absorbing the anxiety and uncertainty and frustration, leaving them free to focus on their screens. 'Where was your husband?' I ask. 'Oh, I don't know really. Panicking a bit. Getting cross with me because I didn't know what was happening, and I'd planned the itinerary.'

Let me clarify: this is a woman who happens to work longer hours than her husband, who, for medical reasons, had needed to 'slow down' and was now conveniently victimised. This meant his wife had to 'speed up', and was herself now suffering the medical repercussions of this – namely, raised blood pressure and the whisperings of an irregular heartbeat.

This is also a husband who expects his wife to cook separately for him, in order to help manage his condition – essentially, a husband who has allowed himself to become another dependent on her. He knew at some level he should be taking adult responsibility on the trip, and was panicking because he was now looking somewhat unmasculine. Why do we feel we need to look after men in this way? To save them from their own uncomfortable feelings? Oh yes, just rewind back to the classroom – sit next to this little boy and *steer him*, please!

This husband was afraid to step up for fear a temporary co-parenting role slip into something more permanent. He was therefore irritable and confused: 'I need to look in control right now! I don't know anything about the situation! I don't want to be in control of it because that spells work. But I should look more in control! How can I look in control? You're failing to provide me with the means to look in control, woman!'

As Adult Women become more ostensibly 'in control' and capable, and begin to pay for more of the domestic outgoings – cleaning, holidays, childcare – men can feel impotent and insecure. They're no longer able to crow, 'I work these hours so I can pay *for your life*!' They need somewhere to put this anxiety. From what I see in clinic, they frequently take it back out on their partners, who they see as holding on to some form of power, which deprives them of theirs. And frightened men are often aggressive men. He externalises his feelings as a way of defending himself. Since men are typically taught that to be emotionally open is to be vulnerable, he prefers to locate that vulnerability in his female counterpart. He *projects* it. In turn, the confused woman tucks away her feelings at his attack – spelling detrimental impact to her well-being. She *suppresses* her rage, and the internal conflict of this certainly elevates cortisol, which creates the perfect environment for bodily expression.

In Adult Womanhood, it's not just family life where we see our rage stirred and squashed; society has myriad ways of placing its impossible demands on us too – for example, through childlessness. We know all too well that our position is vastly complicated in very many opposing ways when we don't have children, whether by choice or not. My patient Bianca is a case in point. In Bianca's life, her mother-in-law was the mouthpiece for society's judgement. I've found that most patients with 'mother-in-law' problems report them arriving at the point of having – or not having – children. This is where values and world views really seem to clash, and we're often up against quite outmoded ideas that arrive with force and criticism.

Bianca
Anger as fibromyalgia. Her strategy = Physical aggression

Bianca was not able to have children. When we first met, she was processing the indescribable pain this caused her and, over the ensuing years, used therapy to work out how to move forward with her life. When she arrived in my consulting room, Bianca had recently been diagnosed with fibromyalgia. She attributed its onset with the discovery that she wouldn't have children. 'A week later, I couldn't get out of bed.' Across the course of our work together, Bianca exhaustively explored the different roads available to her and her husband. She just didn't feel she could subject herself to the anguish of IVF, since her sister had gone through hell on that journey. She felt her body would not cope with further intervention or assault.

The couple explored adoption, but felt so defeated by the red tape and obstacles they just didn't feel they had the strength. Their shared emotional landscape had been completely torn apart by this news. To intensify matters, there was a cruel and insensitive mother-in-law (MIL). MIL emerged not just from a different era, but a different class and cultural background to Bianca. She was cosseted, selfish and deeply unempathic. She was materialistic and exclusively concerned with family reputation. 'She doesn't even *like* children! They were all reared by nannies and packed off to boarding school by the age of seven!' Bianca cried.

Therapy was painful, and Bianca had to contend with an emotionally stunted husband and his mother whispering in his ear. She was convinced that MIL was sowing seeds of mutiny and that her husband would jump ship for someone able to provide him with a child. MIL herself was anti-adoption, which was in fact part of the psychological red tape. Her influential whispers can only really be described as fascistic, and based on her desire for an heir to exhibit purity of lineage. Bianca was on her knees and close to complete defeat.

Together, week by week, I emotionally bottle-fed strength to Bianca, as you might a baby lamb. She was initially so defensive of her husband and his family that I had to gain her trust before handing her the goggles. When Bianca was able to tentatively glimpse through them, they would ultimately reveal the tangled mass of human vipers writhing around her. By increments, she began to understand their nastiness and mal-intent forcing their way into her.

Initially, Bianca began to venture information about the horrifying things MIL had said to her, to do with her body and, by implication, how it was letting her down. That perhaps this had something to do with her generally flawed genetics. Because MIL's dagger-throwing came via 'apparently innocent' questions, it left Bianca muddled and confused about what she sensed she was witnessing. As I helped clarify the real meaning of the interrogation, and the penny dropped for Bianca, she became more emboldened.

Prior to one weekend visit from her husband's family, I encouraged Bianca to take herself up to the bedroom when the attacks began (they would always be brilliantly timed so that Bianca and MIL were on their own in a room together) and use her husband's tennis racket to pummel the mattress. This proved an absolutely pivotal moment in our work together. From this time on, with more humour and outwardly verbalised aggression in her sessions,

Bianca was able to access her anger. Her body slowly began to repair too.

It happened so incrementally that this was imperceptible, until the day I noticed she wasn't hobbling and stood up from the chair with ease. It turned out that not only was she smashing up the mattress when the MIL came to stay, she was doing it regularly throughout a day. 'It's important to me that I start and end a day with violence,' Bianca said, before we both laughed at this brilliant logic. 'That's not something you hear women saying nearly enough,' I tittered.

What was wonderful, in terms of Bianca's continued recovery, was the application of this released energy into her language. She now didn't need to leave the room and rush upstairs for her racket when MIL uttered an abhorrence. Now, using the words forged in our work, in combination with the rage she had clearer access to, Bianca began to release her feelings in the moment. Using language. Powerful, choice language. Sometimes accompanied by covert 'push-away' hand movements, which distilled the energy of the tennis racket, and near-perfectly encapsulated her emotions. She called the racism what it was. MIL found herself shocked. And, importantly, silenced into reflection.

Bianca's story illustrates how little choice women have *but* to internalise the crushing forces of need and demand in their environment. But this also goes for MILs, who themselves are forged within the frying pan of the social conditioning they've been subject to. Society does this to all of us – and then pits us against each other, as we try to crawl through the quagmire of various conditioning. The patriarchy helps create a battleground for women, rather than a neutral pitch on which ordinary ideas can be batted about. If we were able to have straightforward conversations with those who are labelled enemy, all of the energy spent on hating behind backs and trying to wade through projections and perceived projections could be put to different use. Which, you could argue, is why society prefers that we stay wrapped up in conflict with each other – because, that way, we're not muscling in on the real action.

Having said this, the topic of in-laws frequently arises. Adult Woman seems to find it difficult to say what she really feels, for fear of seeming ungrateful or impolite. When we get down to the brass tacks of her view on how she's being treated by MIL, it transpires that it's mostly rage. Adult Women patients divulge that, when it comes to the relationship with his mother, you can't win. You're a threat, you're the Other. And yet you feel a pull to impress and be the most desirable daughter-in-law, forcing you to swallow those feelings of anger. Although you're really the one in the power position, you expose yourself through fawning. How did these MILs become so hardened towards the younger versions of themselves? Could it be that there's no other way of expressing the inequities of their own lives than towards this subsequent generation, who has *so much* to be grateful for?

Women patients have hinted at feelings of uncomfortable envy emanating from their MILs, a feeling that she's taken something which she doesn't have a right to. There's a strange fact which might contribute to this – microchimerism. This is when cells are trafficked between mother and foetus in pregnancy. Male DNA has been identified in the female brain, suggesting that little bits of her son are lodged permanently in the brain of his mother. Gross but true. This has implications for her body as it ages, in terms of certain vulnerabilities to disease. Perhaps MIL feels, at some fleshly level, that her body has suffered to produce him, whilst his partner just waltzes off with the spoils.

Here we have two women suffering in different ways, and one man: oblivious. Look at the complexities, conscious and unconscious, we're grappling with here. My bafflement grows, year on year, at this assumption that, as Adult Women, we're meant to step up and provide care for families throwing so much at us. I missed the bit where we agreed to this. And yet, most of us unfailingly oblige, not questioning the new reality that, though these relationships might have made us suffer all our lives, here we still are, showing up for duty. What the *actual* …? Can you imagine if we started refusing? How long before civilised society collapsed? And why do we find ourselves outlandishly celebrating the men who volunteer for a school trip or give someone a birthday card (often, in both cases, because they've been encouraged by a female partner, let's be honest)? Doesn't this underscore just how incapable we've all allowed men to become?

Something of this sense of *doing extra, going further, no questions asked*, does prey on a vulnerability which gets wired into women: that tendency for second-guessing the needs of another; the thoughtfulness and empathy which we're conditioned in, and which mothering naturally exploits.

This makes it difficult when society takes it one step further by relying on women to take up these responsibilities. Which in turn makes our professional life harder. As Adult Women, we're also trying to be taken seriously at work. Whilst moves towards equality and diversity are shouted about loudly by many employers, from what I hear, the reality doesn't often match up to the lip service. School receptionists apparently find themselves as equally hardwired into the patriarchy. It's the mother who's subjected to the scornful phone call for forgetting to pack a PE kit or the ingredients for a home economics class; the mother who carries the primary guilt of missing an assembly or a sports day. Perversely, it's also the mother who misses the promotions and faces streamlining and redundancy drives, and doesn't have much of a leg to stand on, when those around her are able to appear so easily committed and unconstrained. And if it's not the facts of her life per se, tripping her up professionally, it's the ill health caused by trying to conceal the chaos. On the subject of promotions, it feels necessary to add something about the old boys' convention of golf courses and football pitches, Lycra-clad cycle rides and gentlemen's clubs. This BS is still happening – and, listening to my patients, it's just as prevalent as ever. Yes, we might pity men that they can seemingly only communicate through talk of leagues and handicaps. But we shouldn't. This is the territory where deals are sealed, allegiances drawn and professional advancement guaranteed. Discrimination is real, ladies. And they're not letting you see it.

Let's hear Anika's take. Anika is your best friend, your sister, your cousin. She's you. She's every crushed woman trying her best to grapple with all of the above and then some.

Anika
Anger as panic disorder. Her strategy = Music and 'embarrassing running'

Anika is a designer who suffers with mind-bending panic disorder. She calculates she's lost years of work to it and countless promotions. At the beginning of therapy, Anika's long-term relationship had just ended and she was attempting to acclimate herself and her eight-year-old daughter to life within a single-parent household. She would sit with a frozen expression in our early sessions, detailing how the anxiety would start low down in her spine and 'all of a sudden be up on her chest'. It caused a paralysed sensation, resulting in her gasping for breath and running, sweating, towards nearest exits. Worst of all, the experiences recently had sometimes begun to end in dissociation, where her mind appeared to 'separate from her brain' and float above her. She would watch herself from the outside and struggle to reconnect with herself.

These states can perpetuate, because if our brain has experienced what it reads as trauma, dissociation can be identified as a self-protective solution. Fortunately, because Anika had only recently begun to suffer in this way, I knew that 'wiring back' could be established quite quickly. If you've ever dissociated in anxious states, you know how horrible it is. But the treatment isn't magical or wishful thinking. It's a question of patient, dedicated retraining – and doing something else with the rage.

Anika and I got straight on to a programme of

reteaching, principally involving dance and music. Anika proceeded to put on uplifting pop tunes at home, in the car or at work. Ambient sounds were better than those piped in through headphones, which could lead to distancing and disorientation. And she began to dance. A lot. Furiously, angrily; characterised by outrageous moves and giddy laughter. I encouraged laughter as much as possible. She'd reported a 'pit' in her stomach, which people suffering with panic mention quite a lot. Since 95 per cent of serotonin is produced in the gut, it makes sense that this is where the hollow is felt. I advise patients to reinterpret their distressed, panicky feelings as excitement – since they involve the same hormones of cortisol and adrenaline – and, invariably, a different relationship with their symptom is quickly established.

Indeed, after three weeks, Anika reported some positive results. The frequent 'embarrassing' runs I'd prescribed, which caused her daughter no end of shame – and involved Anika throwing her arms around manically and whooping intermittently – were having an impact. As were the intensive 'home music therapy' sessions. Anika felt that her panic attacks were changing form; that she was starting to feel ownership of them.

This allowed us to focus more intently on the cause. Anika had been the academically successful youngest child of a family with two disabled older brothers. She was both the beacon of light and the emotional crutch her parents lent on for proof that they hadn't 'messed everything up'. The sentiment was cruel and cold, and the emotions behind it were desperate and dripping with unspoken fury and resentment.

Anika bore the mantle of responsibility daily, whether by helping actively with her brothers' care or, as her working life took off, by offering support remotely to her parents via hours-long evening calls. The problem was, this role of caregiver had teed her up for a marriage where she was recruited into the same role.

Anika is still in therapy, three years on, with no intention of leaving – knowing that she needs to keep her daughter safe from the intergenerational attacks which could land on her. Anika is still discovering her story, as for so many years it was written by other people. The multiple flavours of anger this has left her with are tangible. Some days in her sessions she shouts, in others she cries. Sometimes, she sits shaking her head in horror, seeing herself as she now sees her daughter, and railing at The Load she was expected to carry. She exclusively sees her now-historic panic attacks as cries of fury, with no other outlet available. She always talks to her daughter about anger and the importance of voicing it at the time you feel it, never wanting her to suffer in the same cauterised way she had to.

What Anika's story helps illustrate is that, in spite of the fact that the world looks as if it's carving out a place for women, the reality *feels* very different. Another patient, a social worker, tells me that her in-laws came to look after the baby one day because of a childcare issue. The husband, an IT consultant, returned from work slightly after her. My patient had prepared a roast chicken dinner for them all to eat. After eating, her MIL rose and addressed her: 'Come on, let's do the washing up – *husband* has been at work all day.'

Another patient, working in London's financial district, told me of how she'd passed a younger woman dropping her child off to nursery at 7am that morning. 'She looked perfectly made up. Everything the baby needed was right there, hanging off the loaded-up buggy. But I saw that woman's eyes. She was tired. She looked like she had it all together, but I saw the day ahead in her eyes.'

That same patient had been coming to see me for a number of years, the most of which time had been spent trying to extricate herself from working as a hospital consultant. She was exhausted, and one of her three children often needed time off school for his asthma. But she'd been in a dilemma about leaving a job which she felt defined her and which honoured the work she'd put in since she was herself a Little Girl. Additionally, she wasn't married to her partner (who'd always refused to 'be tied down' – in spite of the fact they'd had three children together). She was frightened of his subtle and slow disdain towards her potentially unemployed self. She was also frightened that, financially, she would put herself in a precarious position.

These stories aren't unusual. Somewhere across a woman's maternity leave, the man shoots ahead and becomes embedded at work. His career then becomes the intractable, the given. The trend that began on maternity leave for her to take responsibility for the home doesn't stop when she returns to work. She ends up doing both. Whilst he's now established as the 'main bread-winner' (though their earnings may not differ substantially), her career is demoted within their partnership, and her dented self-esteem and additional childcare responsibilities mean that she's less able to push herself to the fore at work.

Worse still is the way women end up acclimating to the loss of true equality and partnership in their relationship when babies come along. I hear with strange frequency how, from this point, men start bandying in-vogue terms to denote their objection to curtailment of their freedom. As with Young Woman, I hear they start accusing their wives of 'controlling' and 'gaslighting' behaviours, to demonstrate how irritated they are at being asked to provide information about when they'll be home or whether they can help a bit more. I see women then, in spite of themselves, become placatory and fawning, and try to shrink their needs from view. It feels part of the age-old truth that we are actually frightened of men and what they can do to us. Even our own partners. The ones who made promises to be better than that.

If we're thinking about where violence against women begins (which, to be fair, you might not have been) … this point about having to ask for the basics and realising that even asking isn't helping us – this is where I feel violence gains a foothold. We're already begging, basically.

In the phases of Girl, we see her internalise the need to please. In Little Girl and Teen Girl, we see how she's made to connect with her vulnerability. In Young Woman, the desire to be the Best Version of Her (for him) is cemented. And in Adult Woman, she realises that the choices she faces are impossible and, if things aren't going to feel worse for her, she needs to find ways to suck it up.

The riptide of passive violence is further established via

permitted ineptitude of man-child husbands who forget to tell their wives they're working late or are going for a drink(s) after work, or by becoming expertly panicked at the idea of taking a child to a party or playdate. This indirect brand of aggression is echoed in the pressures placed on Adult Woman by ageing parents and inflexible employers, or when she discovers she's getting paid half the salary her male counterparts receive, in spite of having dedicated her life to the job and even actually foregoing a family. One patient realised recently she'd never be able to afford the same apartment equivalent male colleagues were discussing (because eventually, of course, the pay gap inevitably extends to a complete quality of life opportunity gap).

These moments aggregate across a woman's life, as well as in the unconscious of the men who surround her. There exists a set of expectations which both women and men come to anticipate from their conditioning and from their treatment by employers and wider society. Women become adept at the 'workaround', or learn to magically distort time in order to render themselves visible/invisible as needed and present in all the places she's expected to be. Those around her – children, men and other family members – grow used to the endless services on offer and stop seeing these feats as extraordinary or worthy of gratitude. This subtle denigration and exploitation become evidence of exactly that ordinary, invisible violation of Adult Woman we're talking about.

At what point does 'superwoman' become the mug who's being aggressively taken advantage of? When does the desire to be absolutely the right thing for everybody – colleagues, clients, bosses, children, parents and husbands alike – morph into her becoming the downtrodden object who society has, yet again, pushed into a convenient shape and moulded according to its needs? It's not as if we were genetically encoded to learn how to cut tiny toenails or find an after-school gym club. These *look like* choices, this looks like agency and free, educated will. But don't they ultimately add up to a set of perceptions which fundamentally haven't changed all that much? But because they're now apparently so much more driven by 'choice', if we ask for help with any of them, this incites incredulity. Our feelings of failure then provide ammo to those who seek to exploit or make us feel less-than. A perfectly, quietly violent ecosystem. Women ensure they're submissive – they debase and diminish themselves, and accept the imposter experience to let men feel they're still the boss. Who knows, perhaps what lies on the other side of the patriarchy could be worse? At least here, we know the rules. If we laugh at them, they'll kill us, or at least kill our chances at promotion. Violence is wired into our gendered system.

Rates of gender-based violence globally have actually increased. In 2020, the equivalent of 11 women and girls every minute lost their lives to someone in their family. We also need to remember that half of cases are never reported. Women are somehow still considered the go-to site for expressions of male rage. I feel the repression of our own has something powerful to do with that. If you could sit where I sit, you would have your eyes opened to the number of households in which violence against women is brimming either just under the surface or breaking through into actual physical or sexual harm … You possibly live in one of those households yourself. If boys and girls grow up in households witnessing parity between the sexes, in terms of privilege and power, we'd need to assume it has some impact on the ways these children grow up thinking about and respecting each other. But the boys and girls in our society don't witness equality. They just don't. I was at an 11-year-old's party the other day. Each gender took up their side of the room. It's a given. This happens. Why does it happen? Because *we make it happen*!

I would, at this point, go as far as to term the conventional care model in families abusive, and one which, in its horribly innocuous way, provides fertile ground for more overt forms of violence. I've seen horrendous scenes of marital abuse play out between some of the richest couples in the city. Women who are too frightened and who've waived all of their rights and the financial means to walk away from situations which are, frankly, killing them. And some who are too concerned about their husband's mental states or levels of hatred to leave them alone with children, so are forced to stay put.

For the Adult Women I see, there can appear to be a benefit to turning chameleon and fragmenting the self in multiple, mutable ways. A woman can evolve in her second life after having children – she gains in wisdom, experience. The adoption of new roles forces growth and can electrify confidence. Men are, by contrast, left creatively shrunken and abandoned, which can sadly lead to cruel and subtle ways of enacting their envy. They lash out and inhibit us as a reflex, a bit like a movie villain resurrecting himself in his death throes, following his apparent death.

Such men can become aggressive in passive and cruel ways, envious as they are of a woman's increasing strength and capacity. It takes a different kind of man – an emotionally stronger man, perhaps one who himself has had some therapy

– to allow a woman this opportunity to flourish in her multiple roles, and not feel intimidated and crushed by her growth. Understand that I am speaking about *parts* of a man's mind. It could be that, in their conscious actions, these men are able to congratulate their partner and support her. However, an unconscious part of him is possibly at war with the threat of equality, because it would potentially change his world. It's understandable that this would be scary. Imagine if men could be braver. Imagine if, instead of fighting us, men could say – 'I'll pick that up! I'll sort that washing, make the lunch, take the day off for a sick kid! Forget about my ego, like I expect you to forget yours. We're not at war. This is a partnership. I love you. We are The Team.'

As I hear the same themes in the therapy room spoken of time and again, I wonder whether they capture the ways in which society absorbs male aggression into its steadfast structures – from the pay gap to stuck views of older relatives concerning housework and childcare. These structures then feed the individual male's conviction that it's 'normal' to lap up the offer of professional travel, insist on breakfast meetings and avoid the multiple aspects of looking after growing humans, which women hold in their minds since the earliest days of their maternity leave.

In its turn, society still takes our numb acceptance of this status quo and tailors its marketing and branding and deep economic templates around it. These messages prove very difficult to deprogram from, because they merge and align with those we grew up with, from Girl Baby onwards. Most of us, globally, have been brainwashed by experiences of domestic zones dominated by women, as well as women performing all caring roles, from early years teaching to nursing. When you hear the current generation of Adult Women discussing the backdrop of their young lives, it pretty much sounds just as if second-wave feminism passed it by, in spite of what we were officially taught in school about being able to Have It All. The evidence on the ground just wasn't there. That wasn't being modelled.

So, the expectations of these Adult Women certainly began young, as well as for the men who surround them. But I would strongly argue that we haven't done anything to change the pressures that were on Little Girl back then. She's still recruited to cheer people up, entertain, look beguiling, behave politely as given. Look around you. Society expects more of girls and women in these key areas. Areas which drain and leave diminished energy for other pursuits, whether that be academia, forging an authentic identity or self-care. The messaging remains insidious. It's perpetuated and perpetual. Girls, and then women, do it to each other when they denigrate and run other women down behind their backs, rather than having a playground punch-up and clearing the air quickly. Men do it to us when they don't *insist* on sharing parental leave. And tell us about 'other wives' being benign and accepting. This, by the way, is unforgivable. We can't call them to account, since we don't know these 'other wives'. It pits us against the competitor in a brilliantly efficient move. Gross.

I found myself giggling recently about the apparent absurdity of a Scottish parliamentary apology to women of the 1600s who had lost their lives after having been accused of witchcraft. I thought about it more deeply and wondered, actually, whether things have moved on all that much. A ducking stool was used to ascertain a woman's innocence. If she drowned, she wasn't a witch. Either way, she dies. This sense of being stymied whichever way you turn, of being punished in varying ways for being too successful or too unsuccessful, too present as a mother or too absent, too doting a wife or too needy, hasn't gone away. If you're too honest, you're a bitch. If you're not honest, you're a bitch.

Perhaps that witchy apology was not so misplaced after all. But who's apologising for the crimes of today? Other women happily point the finger, in order to ward it away from themselves. *She's a slag/she's neglecting her kids/look at her cankles.* The fearful side with the bully – 'twas ever thus. We keep ourselves silent for fear of what will happen if we don't.

So we see that violence against Adult Woman comes in many forms, and includes the emotional violence we enact on ourselves, which keeps us tied to a set of behaviours which don't appear deeply different to the Dark Ages.

So, Adult Woman – Parenting … The Load … The Sandwich Years – how can we help you begin to voice your rage when, frankly, you don't have time? Instead, you become a zombie army, controlled by guilt and social pressure into providing a raft of care on behalf of wider family or the government. The aggregate effect of continual self-erasure and suppression takes its toll. This kinetic energy has to go somewhere. The journey from small-scale microaggressions, to coercive control, to overt domestic abuse is etched into us, from bafflement to agony, and not knowing how we got here. Is it any surprise that women are exhausted and 'depressed' or 'anxious'? Or, worse, when the inflammation brought about by perpetually repressing these feelings starts to do long-term damage to our bodies. That neuroendocrine dysregulation brought on by carting extreme negative emotion around internally has been connected with the development of several chronic illnesses, and even earlier mortality.

To grapple with the demands of our position, and the pressures those who are most meant to care can put on us, we need the support of other women our own age. They're the ones who get it. But, as with Tween Girl and Young Woman, they've been acted on in all the same ways. They're also victims in high-power/low-power positions, which doesn't seem helpful for stopping bitching and backbiting. The pressure to achieve perfection in parenting and professional life, particularly in later life childbearing, seems to be immense. The volume of gadgets and podcasts and classes attest to this. Yet sacrifice is everywhere for the women in my practice. 'Part-time working' is all too frequently shorthand for stress and dissatisfaction and low self-worth, a sense of not doing anything well.

Is it really possible for women to strive to be the leaders in society, working alongside men and conferred equal respect? Permitted to earn the larger, more influential sums *without being punished*?

A theme repeated, in various ways, by the women both inside and outside of my practice is how constrained they are by casting and stereotyping. In a world attempting to allow for fluidity of identity, women still seem to be stuck within a narrow set of permissible stereotypes, particularly as they age. The world, it seems, is still not ready for a woman in her fifties to date a younger man. She feels self-conscious about her attraction to men 10 or 20 years her junior, though, of course, men would never have to tolerate this type of shaming ridicule.

The reality remains that, if as a woman you're striving

for respect and a position at the table, you'll need to accept that seeing you there still feels unnatural to many people. If you're daring to aim for positions of potency, whether sexual or professional, you *will* be sniggered at; they will need to denigrate you, to render you ridiculous, even as faintly horrifying. It's the witch again. I'm not saying men are immune to becoming figures of fun or threat, just that we're still light years behind when it comes to allowing women to bend the pre-assigned, pre-decided roles. This is doubtless another roadblock to being able to see ourselves freely, in a way which permits access to pure feeling, unfettered by impotent frustration or even rage. And which makes that path easier to navigate and less threatening.

What we can do for Adult Woman

- Men! Why aren't you also grappling with Having It All? Why is this still something only applicable to your female partners?
- Before we have families, we have to figure this out. As above, if this is when you're planning a family, what will this look like? Who's going to look after the household? What about finances?
- Set up a proper, shared calendar. With reminders. Tech can do some heavy lifting here.
- Male partners! Are you listening? Are you still listening *properly*, after these years of being with her?
- Employers: get with the programme! Why aren't more of you offering shared paternity leave which

enables fathers to live off the income? It looks like 'protection' of mothers who've given birth. It shakes down the same as ever.

- You know all those employment programmes to get women more assertive and able to ask for pay rises? What about training programmes for men, where they're taught how to allow women space and respect?
- Wider families: try to be a bit self-aware. Look at your behaviours, look at what you're choosing to say. If you're not actively trying to be cruel or unhelpful, what's this statement/action in aid of?

Ready to see others glaze over as you walk into the room, finding staring out of the window more scintillating than listening to you? You're ready for the menopause!

CHAPTER TEN

Menopausal Woman

'WHERE HAVE ALL THE WOMEN GONE?' is a repeated refrain across financial districts, the legal sector, senior management roles and exec boards. Er … Maybe they've been called away to a teen in crisis at university? Or have a parent living 100 miles away who has fallen down the stairs? Or maybe their anxiety symptoms have finally overpowered them … According to the UK Parliament's First Report of Session 2022–23 on Menopause and the Workplace it was found that 900,000 women had quit their jobs due to unmanageable experiences of menopause. As with all data gathering, the real statistic will be much higher. Many women don't report or don't see their symptoms as worthy of naming. Nonetheless, employers recognise the brain drain of wisdom and expertise brought about by the mass exodus of, historically, only recently arrived female employees who've responded to a mix of internal and external cues to shuffle off into the wings. As with PND, I'd argue that the 'symptoms of menopause' go far beyond the hormonal and need to address the frequently untenable environmental pressures on women at this point.

In this chapter, we examine more closely the reasons we find it so difficult to take instruction from powerful women. And why 'menopause' is a brilliant way of gently showing us the door, just as we're getting going. Indeed, a male GP once said to a Menopausal Woman patient: 'Don't worry! This is nature's way of letting you slope off into the wings.' Men, obviously, are fed no such cues. Do we assume that, for the men making the decisions, this has to do with sexual selection? They don't find us as decorative, so our function is a bit spent?

Menopausal Woman and Younger Woman don't necessarily enjoy an easy partnership either. This isn't helped by the fabled Queen Bee syndrome, where female bosses are found to treat younger female employees differently. Researchers tend to feel this is potentially connected to the senior colleague's own knowledge of what it took to get them there and their concern that other women *should* commit, or would be capable of committing in this way. We come full circle. Our own care pathways, carefully laid down since childhood, once again scupper us now and somehow still land us with a bad rap. Male bosses would not, I think, seek to protect in this indirect way. Or, if Queen Bee operates from more of a pulling-up-the-drawbridge position, her behaviour is a pretty dismal indictment on how much space women feel society will allocate us.

I invite you to follow the example of my Menopausal Women patients, as they attempt to smash up those limiting narratives and rewrite the script. Let's kick off with Simone.

Simone

Anger as passivity. Her strategy = Recruiting the power of water

Simone had worked her way up in a traditional accountancy firm since arriving as a secretary at 18. She was so good at her job that she'd defied all minimal expectations (not that anyone was really paying much attention – Simone had perfected a way of moving unseen, lest anyone notice her and decide she wasn't up to scratch). Having completed professional exams as part of various workplace schemes, by the second half of her career she 'had somehow persuaded them to let me head up a department.' Simone was quietly capable and seen as a safe pair of hands. Until she hit perimenopause. She'd been keen to avoid the horror stories she'd heard so much about and rushed to get herself onto HRT. She had an intrauterine device (IUD) fitted as part of the treatment. She described to me that there'd been issues from the get-go, as far as the coil was concerned. She'd brought herself to therapy at around that time, as she wanted to get on top of the anxiety which hit her in waves (she thought as a result of her hormonal changes, since she'd never experienced it previously).

Simone's problems with the coil centred around a feeling that she was in desperate need of a pee. When she went running to the toilet, nothing would come out. She began to drive herself quietly crazy trying to figure out whether this was psychological ('I *feel like* I have something painful pressing on my bladder!') or actually a physiological issue. Many women discuss their problems with the coil, whether copper or hormonal. It's seen as a cure-all for many female health problems, from birth control to painful periods to HRT. And, just like the contraceptive pill, it's *brilliant*. It means so many women get to live lives a bit more like ... again, men.

Of course, there might be a wider issue here. Men, from their seat of power, haven't historically covered themselves in glory. Do we really want to *be more man*? There's an argument that, in seeking to adjust our biology and level the playing field, we're perpetuating a self-interested form of living which is ultimately detrimental to ourselves and our environment. By looking to earn as much as men, we drive up house prices, we drive up inflation, we chew ourselves up in a capitalist greed machine. Children lose out and psychological problems get kicked into the next generation ... In reality, I think *this* view plays perfectly into our notoriously polished guilt circuitry. Power, when shared more equally, actually has the capacity to benefit everyone widely. The voiceless have a voice, different stories are told, society organises itself more effectively, economies grow.

Having cleared that up, back to the IUD – one potential equaliser. Because it's such a relatively cheap and effective way of treating a multitude of conditions, and because so many women do get on so well with it, there's a sense of the silver bullet around it. The conversation seems to go something like: 'Ah! We've finally found the plug [literally] to address so many stubborn health complaints of women – and if a woman has an issue with it, it's assumed that it's her issue as "everyone else is using it absolutely fine!"' – which is exactly what Simone experienced. Whether the device had been fitted incorrectly or it somehow didn't gel with her body, she couldn't get a single health professional to really care, or even take much notice. 'They keep looking at me as if I'm crackers! They seem certain it must be in my mind.'

Many women patients report their uncomfortable feelings about being a 'woman of a certain age' in the health system. Her problems are deeply unsexy. Her uterus is basically just really gross and useless, so anything which is offered to help control it at this point is a massive favour. 'Why are you back again? You and your washed-up womb. Have you still got that, then?' Obviously this won't be *all doctors*. But there's an air of dismissal and, if you're awkward to help, a definite sense you're made to feel it.

Clearly, Simone's confidence was wrecked. In trying to address her terror at being knocked over by the potential car crash of menopause and avoid experiencing a life event she feared would result in loss of her position and respect, she was thwarted by the solution offered. The dilemma felt at once so trivial (a tiny piece of plastic sitting invisibly in her uterus) and so huge. When you get nervous, you want to pee. You think you might. For Simone, running from the meetings in which she felt most adrenalized and vulnerable, this was a genuine possibility.

Together, we looked at the presenting problem: Simone feeling as if she had no control over her body –

that her body was being interfered with from the inside
– and that this was exerting an effect on Simone which
diminished her self-worth and sense of standing in her
world. There was also something about the shame of this
which meant it was difficult to walk tall and insist that her
doctor take her seriously.

'What's the worst that could happen?' I asked Simone.

'I wet myself in a presentation.'

'Why can't you get the coil removed?'

'Because then I risk being flooded with out-of-control,
menopausal periods.'

There seemed no way through. But it was clear that
Simone felt entirely alone with the problem and seemingly
not able to share her worries with medical professionals.
Her fear of reporting any kind of personal issue at work
is something I've heard time and again from women, who
are stymied by fears they'll be erased as a response, which
then shuts them down anyway.

Our bodies, always shameful and on the verge of flying
out of socially approved control, stand ready to betray
and embarrass Menopausal Woman in a whole fresh
flavour. The newly arrived redundancy to our physicality,
together with its increased capacity to trip us up, feels
raw and humiliating – the sweats, the dissociative levels
of anxiety, the self-doubt, the difficulty keeping weight
off. It's so cruel in a world which applauds youth and
put-togetherness, whilst clearly simultaneously ravaging
those qualities. What are we allowing for ourselves?
Our bodies are torn apart by a lascivious societal gaze

when we're fertile and torn apart by derision and revulsion once we're not.

In Simone's case, we needed to allow that rage. Specifically, where rage equals the culmination of years spent dedicated to a company that would see her exit *graciously* and not give any trouble. Where rage is the culmination of years spent wearing clothes which de-sexed her and disguised her feminine form in order to be taken seriously. Now those clothes served a different purpose. They were chosen to disguise the shameful ways her body might choose to let her down, in the eyes of an environment dominated by men and women who'd internalised the confident views of a calmly misogynistic system.

'Blow it all open!' I would implore Simone. I'd urge her to open up the rigid, controlled parts of her mind to different possibilities. Of conversation, of viewing herself. These are our *bodies*; they don't have to be our cages. They can be the motorised end products of our mind, instead. The spelt-out parts of us, moving through space, as directed by our brilliant, unstoppable brains.

Simone began to swim. She enrolled in a women's-only gym, and talked about the weightlessness and freedom of feeling her body supported by another body – one on which she could wholly depend. She swam every day after work, and couldn't wait to plunge in and feel herself held *up*, after a day holding herself *in* at the office.

Something started to happen. As Simone allowed herself to be supported by the water, she dared to allow herself to be supported by me. Suddenly, there were two things in her life on which she could depend. The more reliable she understood we were, the water and I, the more her unconscious dared to believe that other objects might be. She booked in to have longer consultations with a named GP she liked. Together, they discovered that repeated urinary tract infections were the source of her problem. They decided the IUD might not be the best thing for her and, together, planned a different package of care. Simone was beginning to trust that depending on others was viable. That to trust could feel safe, and not threatening.

As Simone's fear of incontinence left her, it became possible to forge a different relationship with her changing body. She liked the silky way it felt in water, and appeared to internalise the experience; carrying it with her on solid ground. Her body began to feel more toned, her muscles more in tune with her. She reported feeling more 'coordinated'. Her mind in itself began to follow suit. She was better able to form calm, fluid thoughts in a way which worked in harmony with her instincts. She seemed more cohesive, more integrated. Simone felt a renewed sense of optimism and excitement towards work, as opposed to the dread and negative projections of recent times. She put herself into more visible positions and eventually became a mentor to younger women. In working with herself, in daring to expect that she would be *met with*, Simone developed into a killer package. It was gradual and graceful, and she absolutely shone.

It's been noticeable how much the men around them have struggled with female patients of mine who hold positions of professional authority. Another example is a Menopausal Woman working in a male-dominated tech company who was a manager and requested feedback for her annual peer review. It was damning. One co-worker admitted she did her job well. She 'challenged' her team, which, in some ways, was what they grudgingly admitted they needed. But this was clearly a double-edged sword. She was accused of not being 'caring' enough. Apparently, she wasn't sufficiently empathic. Another colleague stated she hadn't supported him leaving work early to go to his child's assembly. Therefore, he couldn't give her his endorsement. What a reversal of roles.

A woman would scarcely dream of advertising her personal life at work. But in my patient's situation, the man involved was privileged in being provided a platform, a forum through which he could denigrate and expose her for her 'lack of empathy'. When I asked whether she thought they'd punish a man who exhibited lack of empathy, she had to admit, no they probably wouldn't. These would be 'weird' things to accuse a man of. When I then asked whether she'd consider bringing this observation to her appraisal, she was horrified. 'Accuse them of sexism? They'd never forgive me. No, I couldn't do that. They'd find a way to get rid of me. I'd be like a bomb going off. No.' So she quietly seethed, now that the goggles were off. But, over time, the knowledge that someone else had seen and named the sexist treatment, that there was a reason for this feeling, emboldened her. She no longer heeded the passive aggression of these particular employees. She didn't feel confused about the impotent feelings it stirred in her anymore.

She knew what they were doing, which meant that a new form of emancipation was actually possible, because their attack was no longer hidden. She found a couple of other female co-workers dotted about the firm. She shared her experiences, and they shared theirs. They're now making plans about the changes they're going to insist on.

It sounds so obvious when stated out loud – that, of course, these men, cosy in their male-heavy environment, would be disinclined towards a woman intruding and upsetting the order of things. But, as women, we're loath now to admit we might be locked into these hackneyed old scripts, too. We'd believed we were liberated beyond this. Sadly, I think this myth of liberation leaves us more exposed.

As another example of women being hoisted by their own petard, another Menopausal Woman patient worried about the 'Me Too' movement and whether ultimately it would make men too afraid to hire women. Her concern was that, by bringing women into roles of influence in the workplace, men can feel they're juggling a hot potato, which leaves *them* afraid to speak – the double bind for women of being frightened to call out the thing you know everyone fears you'll call out. We bias against ourselves. *I am the bomb*, as my tech patient worried. Being afraid of upsetting us creates a self-consciousness in men which adds to their own sense of frustration, and who are they likely to take this out on? They've never had to feel self-conscious before. *Who's making this happen*? Her, the witch! Burn her!

As a point of habit, I encourage women to ask themselves, would this happen to a man? This can alert us to the number of situations in which we're blind to casual sexism. It applies to the male jogger in the park who barks at you to 'get out the way', the dad who wouldn't let you drive his car because you're 'too short', the female boss who doesn't employ mothers, the patronising mechanic or plumber or electrician or doctor. You know it, you feel this daily.

You may also be smarting from the accusation that 'home working', popularised by the pandemic, doesn't work; perhaps because you're a woman, who's recognised an increase in her productivity as a result of not commuting, being on hand to resolve small domestic demands which, ordinarily, you'd need to shoot home or make stealth phone calls to resolve. In my experience, it seems that men struggle more when trying to work at home. A domestic setting signals disruption and multitasking. So perhaps it's no accident that the loudest voices calling for full-time office return seem to be male. 'It's not possible to be as efficient from home!' Not *for you*, maybe …

If we can start to identify these insidious but influential notions and behaviours as *sexism* (even if just in conversation with ourselves), a lot of the anger building behind the scenes starts to resolve. Gradually we begin to talk about it openly again, and slowly the narrative surfaces. We need a new wave of feminism. One which men feel is theirs too. If they've been asked to assess whether they can Have It All, if they've been brought into this idea from the get-go, then we're suddenly talking about a *people*ism. We need to wake up to all of the patterns we've sleepwalked into. It's as if every time something new comes along (jobs in tech, homeworking, Me Too), we tend towards slotting ourselves into a place of oppression next to it instead of seeing it as something which could help us. The consequence being? *It's making us ill.*

We only have to look to the examples around us of women

struggling to succeed 'at the top'. I won't name names, since this will date the point too quickly; for every name I now use, another will come along and replace it. This is an ever-changing roster. Yes, we've had female prime ministers in the UK. Their femininity was an issue. These women were too stiff, awkward. Manly? But also found to be taking *too much* of an interest in clothes. One was reduced to a pair of legs in a too-expensive outfit. Another did everything she could to convince of her masculinity – deepen her voice, take milk away from infants, start a war. It was ultimately too confronting to the men in her party. Mother had to be killed off. In as humiliating a way as possible. Plenty of men in politics are cruel, but they're seen as decisive and focused. We can't take similar from a woman. It becomes evil when a woman is doing it because she should know better, her biology should make her behave differently. It's not only unforgiveable, it is *doubly* unforgiveable.

This strikes a similar note to the women in roles of leadership and authority I work with clinically, who report feeling squashed by pressures to be so much to so many, and still feel they haven't 'won'. From the other side, it can look as if females in positions of seniority seem impelled to treat other women badly; patronising, bullying and frequently unsupportive of mothers, denigrated by their male colleagues and subordinates, and reviled by women employees. It's lonely at the top.

It seems to help my female patients to talk through why a female boss might be acting *against* them like this. They use the processing opportunity therapy provides to consider new ways of approaching her, so that different conversations might be established. I'm not saying it's a magic bullet, but I am saying that we mustn't stop trying. The more it's discussed and recognised, the more hope grows that we can do things differently.

That same framework of impossibility impacting female leaders can be applied to most women in the public eye, including those who've found themselves there by horrible twists of fate. Women who've been used as pawns in a man's world and who find themselves doubly punished by a media and braying public who troll her, as if somehow she had a choice. Or female experts who try to go public with their message. Watch out. You *will* be branded a witch, one way or another. Don't get me started on female celebrities. We *adore* them, we *loathe* them. We punish them to point of destruction for daring to claim the attention. Women's outrage at reality is the only way real change can embed, the only way we can protect future generations from the witch-hunt.

An attempt to cut Menopausal Woman down to size, because she isn't feminine enough anymore, is in itself an act of violence. The way my patients feel diminished and humiliated into silence feels equally violent. Their potential isn't reached and everyone's secret hunches are confirmed. The surveys attempting to find out 'Where did all the women go?' appear to convey some kind of shock around the disappearance of so many of the talented workforce. But I think we know the answer. My patient Mara certainly felt convinced of it.

Mara
Anger as cancer. Her strategy = Sleep

Mara maintained that her job had given her breast cancer. She worked as a nurse and was convinced it had attacked her health. The shift-working patterns, combined with the worsening stress of the role, of being afraid that her tiredness levels would result in her making a fatal error, resulted in a rage in her, which she felt had caused disease. Mara was furious that a job she'd committed her life to was now her undoing. At this point in her life, Mara felt that her good nature and eagerness to please had been exploited. She was sure that, looking around her, the lives of her closest friends also bore the hallmarks of, as she put it, 'giving them ourselves'.

Mara needed to find a way of expressing the rage she felt towards her employer. She could name it, but couldn't do anything productive with it. She was convinced that the feeling was being reabsorbed into her body. As we saw earlier, inflammation is linked to chronic levels of anger. A 2021 article in the journal *Nature* found that around 20 per cent of human cancers are associated with prolonged inflammation. The authors propose that inflammation is related to each stage of cancer progression, as well as development of malignancy. It also provides a favourable environment for tumour formation and metastasis. For example, chronic inflammatory bowel diseases, such as ulcerative colitis, carry an increased risk of colon cancer.

MENOPAUSAL WOMAN

Copious studies discuss exceptionally low levels of anger amongst cancer patients, leading to the conclusion amongst researchers that anger is being repressed. Significant evidence also points to suppressed anger as a forerunner to cancer, as well as a component in the advancement of cancer, following its onset. It's difficult to research the relationship between anger and cancer, since you can only survey patients who now *have* cancer, unless you embark on some enormous longitudinal anger survey of the population, and see who ends up with a diagnosis. And if you ask patients who have a diagnosis of cancer currently, you're bound to hear some angry responses. Nonetheless, Mara was convinced, and I've now worked with several women who feel their cancer diagnoses are connected to repressed feelings; most notably rage. Mara ventured that the strain of her schedule and working nights had wreaked havoc with her biorhythms, but felt that her decision to pursue this career was symptomatic of a lifetime spent serving others. She'd arrived at a point where she could no longer work out whether she'd chosen the job or whether it had chosen her. She was beginning to understand the depth of her fury at this possibility. That this repressed reality might have jeopardised her health created a vortex of feeling which was both overwhelming and palpable.

Mara, a Menopausal Woman, had always had difficulty saying no. She'd forever prioritised The Other – from patients to family members to friends – and this hit to her health felt like a clear signal to put up some real boundaries. 'I've heard of boundaries ...' Mara murmured wistfully. 'But I don't know what they look like.' Most women don't. As part of our conditioning, we're very much dissuaded from asserting our needs in the form of lines in the sand. It's really only by beginning to tune in to our emotional apparatus that we gauge enough data to work out what that hard line is.

It's my enduring wish that we take this apparatus – the 'affect system' – as seriously as we do any other system of the human body (we'll talk more about this in Chapter Twelve). Medical science is nowadays vocal about its findings concerning the feedback relationship between brain and gut, between mind and body. Psychoanalysts have known this forever. Freud's famous cases of patients 'somatising', or wearing their psychic pain as physical conditions, are pillars of a therapy training.

Mara needed to start looking after her own body, just as she looked after those of her patients and family. Together, we began to think about ways she could focus on her well-being, so her rage might be satisfied that change was afoot. In therapy, Mara had a place to externalise those emotions, but at home and around work, what did she need to start feeling better? What did she need that she hadn't been giving herself?

'Sleep' was Mara's response. It turned out that, ever since she'd had children, she hadn't slept for more than a few hours at a time. That she would often just get to sleep when her alarm would ring for work. That she'd try to grab a nap when she got back from a night shift, but that the sunlight would keep her awake. She'd eventually give up and survive the rest of the day on caffeine.

Mara was now off work for treatment and receiving statutory sick pay. We decided she would learn how to sleep. Results from scientific studies suggest a robust association between sleep deprivation and mood, based on the fact that the amygdala is implicated in both. Some go further and link anger specifically to lack of sleep. Mara began to notice when she was naturally tired (the cancer treatment certainly contributed to this) and tried to let herself go with these sensations. It might sound basic, but I would wager that most women are running on some sort of sleep deprivation, a problem which definitely worsens for many around the time of menopause. Women fantasise about bowing out of their intense roles at work because they're just so damn tired. Some actually do.

With sleep as her only homework, Mara herself eventually began to settle into longer stretches at night. Sometimes she felt too ropey to come to therapy in person, and we'd have an online session. But over months, and as her treatment came to an end, Mara vowed to stick to her sleep habits. She even negotiated with work to no longer work night shifts. She was finally listening to the boundaries her body had been trying to lay down for her and using them to shape a life which would align with those.

Mara offers us all a salutary lesson. We're reminded by her experiences of how, even at a basic level, everything from our moods, to our immune systems are compromised when we don't sleep well, and the extent to which these fundamentals are essential for well-being. We need to sleep for our bodies to deal with inflammation, and we also need it for our emotional immunity. I talk a lot with patients about this idea. At certain points in our lives, we can all be vulnerable at this level. Our psychological biome can wear thin. Boundaries are more difficult to enforce. Our physical health begins to suffer, which in turn affects our psychology – again, the inextricable link between body and mind. It's essential that we tune in and recognise our personal alarm bells. Whether that's feeling more thin-skinned towards others' behaviours, more antagonised or just emotionally uncomfortable, listen to what your body is telling you. Respect these messages. We can save ourselves from greater harm or damage, emotionally and ultimately physically, when we catch feelings early. Part of this tuning in needs to help us identify where society has laid its tripwires. We need to be realistic about how well concealed they can be. And how the choices we *thought* we'd made about our lives may be examples of this.

Patriarchal structures have woken up to the potential of losing their stranglehold, and seize the opportunity to denigrate and squash wherever they can. Misogyny feels threatened at new levels, so it must devise cleverer ways to retain its internalised triumph. It seems intolerable that women could find their way to the top of their sector. It flies in the face of what we've grown up with. There obviously hasn't yet been a clear and entire generation of women working in an equal way to men, be that in pay or in freedom. By which I mean, freedom to grow with their professional life unencumbered by the demands of the domestic or the structures of the workplace. Both the home sphere and the professional are contingent on each other's disavowal of women as equal. No wonder we're angry.

It feels fitting in this section, where women sticking their necks out results in being killed off, that I discuss how hard it was to write this book. As I mentioned right at the start, I was angry. I was outraged by what I was hearing and seeing. The incoming 'data' regarding the poor treatment of women and their associated ill health just had to be made known. I couldn't not share it – it wouldn't be ethical. But for all that emotion, with every sentence that charged from my fingers, I was filled with an equal and opposite sense of doubt.

I wondered a lot if your 'typical man' would harbour these same doubts. Who is he, anyway? Someone who hasn't had to navigate the daily onslaught, the instructions, the grind, the passive and aggressive signals to get back in the box? But the men I know are beautiful. They're kind, they're confused, they are scared too. OK, I've known some giant shits as well. We all have. We've worked for them. We might have been brought up by them. We've been groped and assaulted by them. But then you have our sons and grandsons and nephews, in all their complexity and promise. I'm talking about a *system* here. A system designed and constructed and upheld by men for millennia. Whose values and institutions can't find a way of truly letting women in. And, sadly, how that system steers us *all*, and gets in, and causes such damage.

I don't think the answer is, 'Do it like a man!' Our knowledge that we're *not* that confident-seeming stereotype of the imagined man after all would erode our *actual* internal strength. Think about the female prime ministers ... Kicked out of the club, ultimately. Her efforts to fit in didn't address the problems of the system. Trying to be masculine denies our real resources, which are multiple and impressive. One of the ways our anger increases is by curtailing these. We need to find our power organically, and then be permitted to express it.

But in taking up my voice in society, it's me as a woman who's scared. Frightened of the cancelling; frightened of the trolling – the safely anonymous hand who can tear you down and finish you off. The attack is planted within us. Our lack of self-confidence and fear mean that we allow the anger to build and destroy us from within. The bomb's already gone off. The weapon is autoimmune. Sometimes our emotional immunity starts attacking the healthy tissue, as well as the diseased. As a therapist, I've always encouraged the reinforcement and strengthening of the good, strong, healthy parts of the ego. If these are bolstered, there's more in the arsenal to handle the unhealthy, attacking invasions to our well-being.

Women are envied and abused for their strength and capacity. This is where the abuse begins. When someone suspects another has equal or greater power, they suppress. Women *do* have greater capacity. Look at what their bodies can do. What happens when you're capable *and* suppressed? You *rage*. As well as what our bodies are capable of, they also challenge us, from menstruation to morning sickness. But perhaps our strength comes in part from the adversity, from knowing what we're capable of handling.

As we mature, we become freer of the need to attract men in the same grateful, fawning ways. We're not subject to the same type of lecherous, denigrating attention. Meaning that we have, in some sense, greater choice when it comes to where we spend our desire. For Menopausal Woman, our life drive can be more for us. Female desire is complex, and has for so much of our life been siphoned through the male gaze. How much of it was ever our own? At this point, as we enter a time post-fertility, where we might dare to take more ownership of our bodies outside of public scrutiny, where do we choose to focus?

Something significant is definitely beginning to stir in the Menopausal Woman camp. Partially, I think there's far less of a fuck given about what women feel about their actions or decisions by this stage, which is clearly pretty liberating. But I also think certain female celebrities have had an enormously positive impact. They've spoken loudly and clearly about what women should expect for themselves and, in various ways, which I've heard repeated back to me by patients, have inspired ordinary people to hold up their heads and fight for what they're due.

Certain GPs are still sending women away with all sorts of alternative diagnoses for menopausal and perimenopausal symptoms, from depression to psychosis. Some still insist on testing hormone levels, which we know is not useful, since levels constantly fluctuate. But trained, patient-centred doctors know that menopause comes in so many different shades of symptom, it's just not possible to apply a one-size-fits-all chemical template. It's not possible to pin menopause down to a hormone level. To try forms part of the same distressing drive to separate brain and mind from body and chemical, and organs and hormone levels from emotion. For heaven's sake, just look at and listen to the *whole* patient. She knows her body better than anyone. She's been in it for 40+ years!

Patti was a Menopausal Women who needed to be put back in touch with her body, which had been trying to tell her the truth for a long time.

Patti
Anger as worry. Her strategy = Bi-lateral processing e.g. walking!

Patti was her mum's full-time carer. She had three sons – lovely, helpful boys who were all variously dotted about the country. They'd come and visit, but Patti did find herself alone with her mum quite a lot of the time. She had lots of friends, but her mum took up much of her time. She was softly-spoken and angelically kind, the sort of person who would do anything for anyone and frequently did. She was always running favours for people and buying little gifts. Even for me.

Patti's husband had left her for a younger woman he worked with. She didn't even sound bitter as she described that time, but spoke of a really painful rash that had developed on her torso. It would still flare up when she felt particularly stressed, and she would sometimes rub that area in sessions, with a pained look. Her worry for others literally 'got under her skin'.

We realised quickly that Patti did nothing for herself. Ever. But that she got a lot of peace from walking – even short distances to the shop or taking her mum for a stroll in her wheelchair. Patti spoke of how it allowed her to clear her head, and she frequently felt more relaxed afterwards. Evidence is established that long-distance walking can ease psychological distress, and we know that the bilateral movement of walking is emotionally reparative. Research points to a reduction in amygdala activity even after an hour's walking. I shared these ideas with Patti and we discussed the possibility of her finding the time to walk for longer distances. Cautiously, she arranged for her mum to go to a day centre once a week, and tentatively planned a proper hike with friends. Patti's anxiety levels surged as we got closer to the date, and worry for her mum increased. We talked about this. I observed that she was a touch cross with me for encouraging the plan and we saw how the relationship between anger and worry formed. She'd begun by feeling affronted that I could have suggested such an outrageous plan, then diverted it almost immediately into worry for someone else, thus sparing me (and herself) from her terrible feeling.

I observed that maybe it had been easier to be a 'worried' person than an angry one. She realised that, when her husband had left, she would channel her feelings into her sons and how they were coping, which concretised into a general concern for them as they grew older. She admitted she found herself far more anxious about them than any of her friends seemed about their kids. As they grew up and moved away, this in turn extended itself to concern for her mum.

As we spoke together across months, Patti got used to exploring her feelings more deeply. She began to recognise just how much she'd blocked them at the point they might register as rage, especially where her ex-husband was concerned. Patti was left shouldering a huge sense of betrayal for all the years she'd believed they were happy, and believed that the things making her happy also made him happy. What began to emerge was a sense that Patti brought care for her mum in to replace the care she'd stopped being able to give her husband. Her feelings of rage were neatly drowned by feelings of concern for her mum, who she'd moved in with. She quietly wondered now if this was for company, as the boys were by that point all at college. Though there was no doubt her mum benefited from having her around, she wasn't so disabled that she couldn't be on her own for a day.

Patti now hikes regularly and is planning a week-long trip with close girlfriends. Her sons eagerly planned between them a schedule of staying with their gran, reportedly delighted that their mum would finally be doing something for herself. Patti walks daily for at least an hour, sometimes with friends, sometimes to meet someone for a coffee. She looks healthy, she has so much to talk about, her horizons have expanded and she calls her ex-husband a 'nasty piece of work' (though she always apologises afterwards). And the rash? Well, she certainly never mentions it.

What we can do for Menopausal Woman

- Start trying to see ourselves clearly. Our identity might have become very blurred. Drill down into feelings to establish who we are at an emotional level, away from others.
- Go walking. A lot. It's great for creativity and it's great for processing painful feelings. And it's free.
- Wear whatever you like.
- Take centre stage. In every possible way you can.
- Support women – younger ones, older ones. This isn't the same as *looking after*.
- Don't spend too long looking back. There are mountains to climb, and you need the energy for that.
- Leave the comfort zone. Every single day.
- HRT, if it's right for you.
- Work life: Claim your space. Life is short. Enjoy the fact that, these days, you seem to care less about what *others* think.

And so, to old age, kicking and screaming and with as little dignity as possible. We didn't bow out when they wanted us to. Damned if we'll do it now. Oh, hang on. I forgot the patriarchy has us by the breasts until we're six feet under.

CHAPTER ELEVEN

Older Woman

THIS IS ARGUABLY a far worse fate than being an old man. For starters, Older Woman is more likely to face neglect and abuse. It seems we go on triggering something intolerable for others, even at this point. Everything we were revered and useful for has left us and, yet, here we *still* are! Taking up space. We're not allowed much, obviously. We're on lower pensions, thanks to the years taken off for child-rearing and/or less well-paid jobs. We're also the ones stuck with enduring either a lonely, cold old age or caring for an ailing husband. Because right now, fulfilling those duties is what's still expected. Older female workers are twice as likely as men to be carers, according to UK Census 2021. A 2022 study clearly demonstrated that caregivers of men were 'more likely to be distressed, remain distressed or become distressed within one year'. The researchers attributed this to older men having more impactive behavioural and health-related issues requiring greater care, and partly because their caregivers are more likely to be younger, healthier female spouses.

WOMEN ARE <u>ANGRY</u>

Distress is an interesting word. It's euphemistic and infinitely pliable. When I speak with older female patients, often with multiple caring duties (which can also include grandchildren), and allow them to properly explore their feelings, what we discover under their apparent 'upset' is a pit of rage and resentment. Yet our entire society is built on 'in sickness and in health' and a denial of any collective responsibility. If she's still standing and can carry a tray, who cares if he's throwing shit at her (literally, in some cases)? These same women might have cared for their own parents or in-laws earlier in their lives, and see this next step as their uncontested due. Interestingly, Older Woman herself is more likely to be denied healthcare, since she's often seen as too fragile to cope with the side effects of treatment. She's also at increased risk of exclusion and poverty in old age.

I've found that, in a more pronounced way than other age groups, Older Woman patients tend not to identify as 'angry'. Instead, the unmet needs of a lifetime become calcified and no longer present themselves internally as hurt or pain. Across a lifespan, those unexpressed feelings seem to decant themselves into an internal crucible, which becomes so full it can bend out of shape. In our old age, the end product shows up as something gnarled and frosty. Behaviours are often so distorted they appear externally as something very different. Friends and family – and even our old-age selves – wouldn't recognise our expressions as anger *per se*. A combination of internal defences and social expectations make it increasingly difficult for us to express the feeling as it exists in its purer form.

Clinically, I've recognised patterns in the expression of anger. Most women seeking therapy are aware that they live in a gendered world. It isn't a surprise to them that a good deal of conditioning has gone into the end product of their feelings. Additionally, we're increasingly bound by socialised rules that seem, once again, to have experienced a resurgence since Victorian times. The Older Women I've worked with are exempt at least from the impact of social media. But its pernicious reach is really just an extension of that historic patriarchal rule-making. Our thoughts and opinions have always been socially policed, which makes the expression of anger or frustration particularly difficult. Nowadays, of course, the threat of being 'cancelled' leaves women even more afraid to voice their views, for fear these are captured and disseminated on spiral.

The harsh kangaroo court of peer opinion isn't new; it hasn't just sprung up since the advent of social media platforms. We've always patrolled our own homes and families for evidence that someone's thinking doesn't align with this week's acceptable ideas. If we've been lucky, we've found ways of working through feelings of anger through conversation, debate and argument, perhaps with blow-ups and heated fall-out as an inevitable by-product. Historically, though, getting stuff aired has never really been typical.

Particularly for women. As a woman, there's always been a lot you mustn't say. You mustn't say you hate your parents, or your MIL, or your male boss. You mustn't say you're angry with the way another woman threw you under the bus. Not to her face. You mustn't say you resent your children or that your ageing father revolts you. Even in the safe space of the therapy room, women couch their thoughts and don't allow themselves free rein to explore and ultimately find a space in which their views might be safely explored or challenged. The threat of judgement feels too dangerous, even here.

WOMEN ARE <u>ANGRY</u>

Working with an older community of women is refreshing, because Older Woman ultimately finds herself a bit freer to say what she feels, keen to experiment with ways of shrugging off the strictures that *she*'s been accustomed to, even if anger itself remains far from her vocabulary. Working with Older Woman also lends a perspective and a certain view back on society, from a lived and possibly quite weary wisdom. She's seen it all come back around three or four times. She's heard the same laments, uttered with new vocabulary, about *apparently* new concepts. But one observation Older Women patients *have* voiced is the extent to which Young Women are now expected to Have It All. My Older Woman patient Suzette's view was, 'It's all very well. But you girls are expected to do *everything*. What about the men? Can't they help?' When reflecting on her granddaughters and great-nieces, Suzette expresses shock that 'There's no support! I had my mother, my aunt, my sisters. You don't have any of that, and yet you're all meant to have wonderful careers. It doesn't make sense to me! There are just all these horrible private nurseries, charging you the earth, whilst the young girls working there sit on their mobile phones!' Suzette on The Eternal Plight of Women was *gold*: 'It seems to take all of your maternity leave to find one which has room! And then you give them your entire pay cheque!' Suzette often simply pointed out The Obvious. Which made The Obvious look instantly mad and ridiculous.

When my Older Women patients talk about their professional roles, if they did have employment outside of the home, it's clear that they were basically paid to *care* – as secretaries or assistants, nurses, sometimes primary school teachers. Although, ostensibly, the roles have different names, the assumption remains that women are the caretakers of the team. Glances angle towards women when a coffee run or sandwich order is needed. Women will be sent for training if their tone is deemed 'too aggressive' and not maternal enough: if you're not great at the soft talk, at the small chat which puts people at ease; if you get straight down to the task, you have some work to do to convince them you're the right fit for their team. Because you're woman-shaped, which ticks a box. But are you *behaving* like one? From what I see, and, sadly, this is backed by global stats, you're either in a low-paid, female-dominated profession or in a profession in which you're lower paid than men. And, somehow, still charged with taking care of them. Be that their feelings, their desires or their digestion.

These assumptions hold domestically, when we're talking about care of older relatives. Apparently it's *natural*, if the woman's been seen as the predominant carer in a family leading up to this moment, that she steps in when people need help as they age or become ill. Why? Just because someone's done it before, are they expected to do it again? The opposite take could be argued: 'Phew! She's really had a run of it. Let's give her some time off now … I know, I'll offer! They're not my parents, but I've known them for 40 years, and they looked after my kids and helped buy our house. *I'll* take them to the shops and hospital appointment!'

Older Woman – having been through the mill and seen it from all sides – can ask clearer questions about her bafflement over the choices of younger women. It doesn't feel so judgemental as when women our own age question us. Older Woman demonstrates her despair for us. Although she had fewer career choices, at least she wasn't left universally grappling, mind and body falling apart, as she also tried to uphold the traditional domestic responsibilities. Let's meet Suzette properly now.

Suzette
Anger as end-of-life agitation. Her strategy = Music. And humming.

Suzette gives great perspective, on everything from careers to friendship: 'Don't fall out with them. Because then they die. And you realise the last word really can be just that.' She described how she'd always been competitive with one of her female friends: 'She even went and *died first!*'

Suzette talked of how we should debate and argue amongst our closest, most trusted woman friends – and not be afraid to, since we very often come to another viewpoint when discussing something which has irritated or confused us. Without this counterpoint, we're deprived of a valuable forum for self-education, enlightenment and development. Working with Suzette was both an educative and terrifying experience. What did I have I to offer her? It turned out, my relative youth, and the opportunity therefore to reflect on her own.

Suzette spoke of how trying to hold her ground at her trailblazing job in news broadcasting in the sixties resulted in her being told she was 'too aggressive, too masculine'. Bizarrely, her granddaughter had been recently told something similar in her own television career.

She was 'too argumentative' and should just 'let things go'. Please.

A familiar tale, this – a workplace still curtailing women because their behaviour needs to fit within a prescribed set of conscious or unconscious expectations, though nowadays, the messaging is more subtle and is often delivered passively, using the language of feminism and female empowerment against us. One woman was told by a highly aggressive man, dressed up as an enlightened art gallerist, that her tone was 'denigrating' and that 'he'd never been made to feel that way'. This patient was mortified. How could she now have become the aggressor? Of course, she hadn't; he just didn't like her holding her ground. This is how misogyny has evolved – to play us at our own game, to know the rules, and use them against us.

Suzette often felt agitated and irritable towards the end of her life, sometimes when reflecting on how little had changed in a world which pretended to be so different. Our sessions were on the phone by this point, as she was in a hospice. Music is a great comfort in palliative care. Suzette began to listen to music constantly through headphones. She talked about how gentle humming soothed and centred her, how the comforting vibrations filled the inside of her body and kept external aggravations out. Suzette would get through entire Nina Simone records without most people noticing. She created an island for herself inside; a calm haven of memories which she didn't have to exert further energy explaining. And then she decided, 'You're all really pissing me off now' and her humming got louder to drown out the world, of which she'd had enough by this point. 'They just think I'm a batty old woman. And they kind of steer clear. Which is just what I want. I want them all to leave me alone so I can die by myself. Peacefully.'

But Suzette liked to use her fading energy to reflect out loud, when she felt someone was properly listening and engaged. It bothered her that her granddaughter was experiencing something so similar, as she too attempted to forge her professional name. Suzette opined that, at least in her day, sexism operated in plain sight. It certainly made her feel pretty distressed to think that, after all she'd fought for and assumed she'd created some influence in, not much had really changed. She even recounted with horror that her great-niece was struggling with a boss who had harassed her and other female colleagues in their large international PR firm. The women were debating whether to take up class action. Suzette seemed to take solace in speaking with a woman (me) who she sensed felt as desperately as she did.

Indeed, on the same day as one of these later sessions with Suzette, I'd spoken with another, Young Woman, patient working in big tech who reported that, however much she proves herself, a white male colleague will always be recognised, promoted and offered opportunities over her. We're evidently even more vulnerable following childbirth. I need too many hands to count the times a woman will arrive speaking of how she's been demoted following a maternity leave or, in some cases, even been made redundant. I've sat with them as they navigate tribunals and complaints procedures; those who can't afford legal representation asking lawyer friends for favours and snippets of advice. I can't say I've ever seen a woman emerge 'triumphant'. She'll sometimes be relieved, sometimes she'll receive compensation. I'd say nothing compensates for the beating her body takes or the battering her mind endures. From where I sit, I'm not sure any amount of money or formal apology undoes this harm. For this is a deep harm – to a woman's self-worth, to everything she was told she should expect. When should she stop trying, if trying results in trying to decipher mountains of legal documents whilst sitting in a milk-soaked T-shirt on two hours' broken sleep and feeling as if everything she's worked for amounts to no more than an insult?

Let's now meet Didi, a patient in her seventies who'd followed a more conventional path than Suzette.

Didi
Anger as overeating. Her strategy = Laughter

Didi was ever the good girl – the sensible, dependable older sister with an emotionally mean father and a mum who didn't intervene to protect her. Didi had always used food to dampen her feelings. She came to see me because she'd lost her appetite. She'd consequently also lost a lot of weight, and said that she wanted to stop hiding; that she only had a limited amount of life left and now felt the need to voice some of the feelings which had surfaced since the food was no longer a mask.

What were those feelings? She'd been docile and well-behaved, had never found a partner and had looked after the father she hated until the end of *his* life. He'd exploited her single status to use her as a domestic skivvy. Her mother had died when Didi was in her late teens, so she'd been recruited as mother-substitute to her two younger siblings. Those younger siblings had left home and moved away as soon as they could. Though they doted on Didi's warmth and generosity, they rarely involved themselves in the life they'd left behind. Cute, overweight Didi had always sorted it. Didi always would. Didi was ever the generous provider: of food, of love, of solutions. And Didi was raging. What to do with this well of feeling which Didi had semi-successfully choked down with food? What to give this woman, so starved of everything she really needed, that food was the only earthly solace available?

Laughter, it turns out. I hadn't planned it, but, in one session, after she'd told me about some particularly brutal thing her father had said to her before he died, she witnessed my jaw drop (I obviously try to hold my feelings back, but, sometimes, you know ...). And an involuntary giggle erupted from her. 'Can you believe it?' she asked, by now shaking her head. 'Can you believe anyone would say something like that to a *dog*? Let alone their own daughter?' I was still speechless, but Didi was crying with agonised laughter.

'He always went for my cooking, which was the one thing I had. The one thing which made me feel capable and I don't know ...'

'Worthwhile?' I offered.

Didi nodded vigorously, tears now streaming as fast as she could frantically mop them. 'He still gobbled it all up. Such a greedy man ... Such a nasty man ...'

Her breathing was coming in fast sobs, but she didn't seek to stem this opportunity for release and recognition. 'And then he obviously went for my size. Such an easy target. This is why no man would want me. He called me The Whale. Since I was eight years old ... And I just took it *all*. What could I do? I would never earn enough for myself to move out – I'd never got my exams. I was completely dependent ...'

The more Didi began to piece together her feelings, the more sessions looked like this. A mix of tears and laughter, a waking-up of emotion, which now spilled from her at a rate she could scarcely control. But Didi became hooked on surfing the emotional cascade. 'Have you heard of Netflix?' she asked me. Apparently, her younger neighbour had shown her how to find it. And she discovered binge-watching. 'I don't binge-eat anymore – I binge-watch!' Ordinarily, you'd need to wonder about the switching of one addiction for another. But Didi had got hooked on comedy: sitcoms, stand-up, slapstick movies – the works. She couldn't get enough. I would try to bring her back to a grounded place in our sessions, but she resisted working more directly with her raw feelings of pure hatred. It seemed laughter made the pill easier to swallow.

In therapy, there's so much thought around needing to be very serious and dig into all the pain and anguish and suffering, so that we can understand it and heal. But, as I mentioned earlier, I've always strongly felt that there's an argument for building up the healthy and 'good' pathways, which protect people as they unearth often very confronting and sometimes intolerable realities about themselves and their pasts. People need to live their lives! They have jobs, families, homes. We don't have the luxury or funds for a complete, Victorian-style unravelling from the luxury of a Swiss sanatorium. An invigoration and reinforcement of the joyful parts of people can help save them from total collapse or regression, which can otherwise happen in therapy, as painful truths surface.

Didi's experiences epitomise the caring demands on women. These demands are even more pronounced for women whose siblings or parents are disabled and for whom becoming the interpreter, go-between or nurse is written more overtly into their destiny. Not only did she 'not ask to be born', to coin an (I think) underused axiom, she certainly *did not ask* to be co-opted into this caretaking role. That role is simply assumed, and similar themes perpetuate through her adult life.

In ways both more and less defined, women *and not men* are in the majority expected, at some point in their lives, to place others' needs before their own. This expectation is something we act into from the youngest possible points, with parents who expect emotional 'kidney-donor' children. That legacy seems to steer us, as we move through our professional lives and beyond. Men might find themselves drawn to helping their parents as they age, but expectation isn't generally carved into their psyche. And unless something absolutely fundamental changes in the way society brings up infants or takes care of old people, it never will be. But, assembling the wisdom of Older Women, it seems that the key reason *Having It All* is *doing us harm* is down to the fact that people are watching us struggle, and seemingly leaving us to it.

Working together, myself and my female patients surface a fountain of fury at our destiny. Once identified, therapy becomes a freeing channel finally permitting women the opportunity to work this demand out of themselves, more able to wrestle away from being hostage to other people's needs. It may not be possible or helpful to confront the people who have 'unwittingly' hurt us, but through the technical means available in therapy (namely, transference and projective mechanisms), we have a shot at feeling a sense of liberation play out. If we can't access therapy, we have to simulate this. The first step is being honest with ourselves about what's been expected of us, and how we feel about that. Then we need to devise means of releasing ourselves from both those feelings and the expectations – and the feelings which lead to those expectations. Right now, these experiences are trapped inside our bodies. Let's get them out. We'll come to *how* in Part Three.

Earlier in the book, there were examples of my female patients using parts of their therapy to reflect on relationships with daughters. A staple for women in their therapy is trying to figure out their relationships with their own mothers. Sometimes issues can become embedded as we get older. Sometimes they can mellow, alongside those who've left us with so much to feel angry about. Justine was someone who still had a lot left to work on with her Older Woman mum, and who ended up having some really raw conversations with her. Arguments, to be honest, which often lasted weeks, and which I was worried might still be in full swing when Justine's mum, Jacquie, died. As witnessed with Teen Girl Katya, a parent dying in the middle of a row isn't going to be helpful at any age.

Justine and Jacquie
Anger as impasse. Her strategy = Asking the questions

Their relationship had always been frosty. Justine had moved abroad to force distance between herself and Jacquie. Justine was an academic, and her relocation to London was just about forgivable on those grounds. Except then, she 'went and married a woman'. Jacquie liked to think of herself as blue-blooded. She maintained she could trace her lineage through to the beheaded French royals. She was a right royal piece of work, as far as Justine was concerned. And Justine had comforted herself that she'd probably never really spend time with her again.

The trouble with this is: our brains don't like it. It's another example of how basic they are, whilst being such simultaneously complex mazes. It was clear how, on some level, Justine smarted with quietly pretending none of it (her mother, her birth, her childhood, her early womanhood, the rows, the threats, the anguish) had ever happened. Something in her just couldn't let her mother go. Don't get me wrong. I've had plenty of patients across the years who've implemented strategic separations – everything from formal annual handshakes to full-blown estrangement. The decision to enact 'divorce' has always come from them. As a therapist, it's beyond my remit to influence that decision. But something about therapy definitely seems to give people permission to look at these relationships in clearer ways. Justine did this, but perhaps not quite how she thought she might.

After realising that she didn't need to justify her decision to put space between her and her mother on my account, it seemed to free up Justine to think in a less angry, rigid way about her. Over the course of months, she shared more about her austere and highly traditional upbringing of 'privilege', which left little room for love and none for affection. She seemed more curious about her mum's own story, and had been left with a few questions. One day, I commented to this effect. And at our next session, Justine surprised me with the news she'd decided to travel to her mum's.

Many of Justine's questions related to the particular pressures placed on her by Jacquie as she grew up. She had been told, 'We are *these kind* of people', 'We do things *this way*', 'What would so and so say if they knew *that*'s what you were doing?' Justine had felt her mother to be a controlling matriarch, whose own life choices were concerned with reputation and family standing. However, as *I*'d asked more questions in the therapy, Justine herself was left asking whether (towards the end of her mother's life) she really knew this woman at all. And whether some of the assumptions she'd made about Jacquie could be blamed quite as cleanly on a foundation of steely nastiness, as she'd long believed.

In fact, through some very honest and upfront questioning (which it surprised Justine to find that Jacquie complied with), some large truths emerged. It turned out that Justine's father had died not of cancer, but of an alcohol-related rupture. Jacquie had been desperate to protect her daughter from the knowledge of his problems, as well as from his debts, which had cost them their home when Justine was six years old. Jacquie had had to work two jobs to support them, as her own parents had long since died, and her husband had spent the money they'd left her.

Clearly, this was a fundamental reworking of the narrative Justine had grown up believing. It wasn't precisely that Jacquie had cleverly curated a cruel personality, in order that Justine wouldn't ask questions. But she had (possibly consciously, possibly unconsciously) chosen to forego a close relationship with her daughter, which protected Justine from the truth and all that may mean for her, whilst inevitably denying her access to a mother who was able to share the robust, generous parts of herself. Those were siphoned off into holding down positions of employment during the sixties. She worked as a secretary

OLDER WOMAN

and as a night cleaner. Justine hadn't known this. Apparently, the elderly insomniac neighbour in the flat next door had padded in and out during the night, checking in on the sleeping Justine. Jacquie was determined that Justine would be protected from knowing about their insecure position. All the reminders of their heritage and aristocratic name at least brought something 'rich' and protective to her daughter. She couldn't give her material wealth, but she could give her this. You can certainly see how rigid and inexplicable Justine would have found this behaviour previously, without the context: the story of a woman trying to survive, and support a child alone, in a world shaped for men, a world which typically would only have made room for women who were attached to a man.

In the case of Justine and Jacquie, finally asking bold questions helped a daughter get to the root of her anger – anger towards her own mother and towards the apparent inability of that mother to provide a proper emotional home for her daughter. Previous to her questioning, Justine had felt cheated of something basic. She now knew it was her father who'd cost her that. For Older Woman Jacquie's part, being able to finally give her daughter her truth meant not dying alone.

Just as our bodies can become repositories of stored anger, so can our relationships. In Older Woman, we see how easy it is to be left with regret, a passive, self-loathing form of rage, and how bitter and compromised it leaves us, to feel hostage to our destiny. It's never too late to rewrite the narrative.

The way this can be achieved is by talking directly back into those relationships which have become receptacles of rage: feuds, fall-outs, family fragmentations … This isn't a manifesto for reuniting families – absolutely not; a lot of them are just hopelessly lost and toxic – but it *is* a reminder to not throw parts of ourselves or experiences we aren't comfortable with back into the gap between us and other people, where they tend to fester.

Just as we can improve the relationship we have with ourselves, and try to use honesty to clarify the channel of our internal conversation, we can absolutely look at applying that same strategy between ourselves and others. Layers of self-consciousness and shame build up around the things we want to say but feel we shouldn't, around the etiquette of what makes others uncomfortable. Where has all of this come from? With Jacquie, there was an idea that something strong and meaningful would be imparted towards her daughter, not through love and transparency about her actual life, but via a fantasy version of a family tree and an apartment in the right arrondissement.

We need to go back and become the limitless child in our relationships, to start communicating from scratch again. Ask the basics: 'Where did I come from?', 'Who are you, Mum?', 'What were your hopes when you had me?', 'What were you excited about?', 'What were you scared of?', 'What made you angry?', 'What makes you angry now?' We assume so much about ourselves and project a lot of those apparent findings onto others, which means we neglect to ask because we think we know the answer.

These assumptions about ourselves are limiting and keep us in boxes of our own making. We assume that we won't be given a promotion, or that we don't have the confidence to ask for more. Could it be that we all too readily accept *less than*, because that's what society has decided for us? That's the assumption society has made. And we internalise it as *our* thinking, *our* feeling. Because of all our conditioning, we lap it up. Because, 'Oh, I wouldn't have the energy to go for that *and* be able to pick up the kids' seems to make a lot of sense. Project yourself forward to Older Woman. What does *she* want for the You of Today? What is *she* telling you to do and say and ask for? How can we avoid sitting with this rage on our death beds; how can we avoid this rage taking us to our death beds? We need to act *now*.

What we can do for Older Woman

- Keep projecting yourself forward to this point and ask yourself: 'Where do I want to be?', 'What do I want to not regret?'
- Ask Older Woman about her own feelings of rage. What would she have changed? What would she advise?
- Do not dismiss Older Woman. Don't make the mistake of writing her off, like the rest of society tries to. You're doing this to your future self, ultimately.
- If you are Older Woman yourself, is there anything you need to tell someone now that you felt too gagged to say when you were younger?
- We need to put the Old together with the Young. Nurseries need to be placed next to nursing homes.

Each has a lot to give the other. We need to keep the thread going and not segregate the life stages.

- Women are still typically the ones recruited to do the dirty work. Enough with being stoic. Enough with protecting others. Let the world know we're wiping bums, and let the world feel embarrassed about it. Say it. Say it all. No inhibitions. No regrets.

Part Three

THE SOLUTION

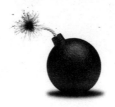

CHAPTER TWELVE

Get It All Out

IN CLINIC, I trace the journey that anger takes through someone's mind, tracking how it lodges itself in these fixed and hostile, yet simultaneously deadening, states. As we've seen, women are fundamentally not permitted their rage. Society and its messaging become absorbed and integrated within our own psychic structure, until we're left so far from our own feelings and instinct as to be completely directed by another set of forces. Our mind becomes frightened of its propensity towards violent thoughts, and converts them in any way possible to render us docile and civil, even if that ultimately compromises our mental and physical health.

We need to get our anger out of all these stuck places and use that energy differently. Our discovery of the relationship between our repressed rage and ill health means that we already have a tool with which to approach our symptoms. Now we can start to recruit other inbuilt resources, in order to understand more of the specifics. Therapists ask questions. They feel for the answers, even the non-verbal ones, with their excellently honed intuition and internal apparatus. We can train ourselves to do something similar and use our own apparatus to challenge our internalised assumptions and defences. Even if therapy isn't possible, this internal toolkit can help to significantly improve our mental and physical health.

Women's Secret Weapon: The Affect System and How to Use It

You'll be familiar with the respiratory and cardiovascular systems. Well, I'd now like to tell you more about the 'affect system', which is the term used in psychology to describe our understanding of emotion and mood. Ordinarily, it's seen as comprising discrete function, like perception or motivation, cognition or behaviour. I would argue that we need to see it as one system with separate but synchronised functions. By tuning in carefully to each aspect of this feelings system, we can use it to our advantage. So many women burst into tears or freeze when they're angry. We need to enable continued functioning of our apparatus whatever the situation, so that it can become a great filter, processor and executor, even without therapy.

This is where borrowing the principles of mindfulness or meditation can really help. We need to get into our internal process, and meditation is a kind of fast hack for that. It's not about becoming incredible at technique, but instead employing the meditation principle as a handy framework for learning to absolutely forefront the *internal*, as opposed to all the chat from outside. It's as if you have two minds in your head: the one *for you* and the one crowded up by the imagined views and feelings of others. I want you to get better at accessing the *you* version, to get better at tuning in. Simply slowly counting your breaths in and out is a speedy way of grounding yourself in the right way. Your thoughts and feelings will try to push their way in. Just keep bringing yourself back to the counting breaths, beginning from one again when you recognise this is happening.

We know that meditation and therapy help regulate our nervous systems. Having a regulated nervous system is vital for the purposes of connecting with our affect system, our emotional circuitry. This system has developed through evolution to be our barometer and guide. In order to help this apparatus best inform our lives, we want to operate within a state of calm and conservation, where energy is spent on 'resting and digesting', as opposed to states in which the sympathetic 'fight or flight' system dominates. The more time we spend in calmer states, the more our bodies are allowed to get on with their own regulation, and the complexities of homeostasis (the stable conditions needed for survival). Once nervous systems are under siege from lots of riled-up *thinking*, the parasympathetic primary tasks controlling resting responses are relegated, and everything leaps to serve the threat of the moment. Persistent time spent in such sympathetic arousal states means our bodies are forced to contend with raised levels of cortisol and adrenaline. This type of flooding means your receptors can become desensitized to cortisol. Unchecked, this can do real damage to our cells and systems, from our immunity to our mental health.

Establish neutral

Because so much of our wiring, from Little Girl onwards, has been about staying out of trouble and being good, we need to be realistic about where that's left us, psychophysiologically. We're conditioned to freeze or shut down when we think we might have upset someone or have done something wrong, which means we're very far from our pure feelings. Society has really kept us away from feeling we might be eligible for anger, frustration, a feeling of offence.

First of all, we need to learn to manage the instinctive flight towards psychological reactivity. We need to reset and refind our neutral so that we're able to get a better, clearer read on what we're *actually* feeling. We need a plan.

Daily plan

Set your alarm ten minutes earlier than your usual waking time. As you're coming into consciousness, kick things off with a really good stretch to get your blood flow going and gently wake up your muscles. Stretching is great for increasing positive emotion, encouraging dynamic interplay between brain activity and the nervous system.

Do a little body scan, starting with your toes and working all the way up. How are you feeling physically? Where in your body are you storing your emotions today? In which ways are you holding them? Don't pick up your phone! Stave that off for as long as you can bear (let's face it, we're all addicted). Keep your eyes closed. Move on to a few minutes of (free) guided mindfulness, focusing on breathing from as low down in your body as possible. Breathe like a baby, from your stomach: you're a primitive being, you're a mammal-baby again. Occupy *this* body on waking.

As you gently get out of bed, try to keep up that lovely deep stomach-breathing. Stretch again, to the ends of your fingertips. Feel every part of you open and gently arrive into itself. We need everything working with us. We need to invite our bodies to be an active part of our decision-making and risk-assessing; we need body and mind integrated and aligned. We're not just a brain in a jar with a few tentacles waggling around or a carefully curated external package with an absolutely neglected nucleus. We're both. All of the time. Avoid the socials until later in the day as they spark off too much extraneous feeling. We need to give ourselves the best shot of arriving into the morning as unencumbered as possible. There'll be so many competing stimuli arriving as the day ticks by. Let yourself have at least this moment.

As you enter into the day, attempt hourly body scans. If you only achieve it a couple of times a day, it's more than you were doing before. We may not be able to give ourselves more *time*, but we can give ourselves more *space*. Again, it's all about learning to approach things from a more internal point of reference. Ask yourself when you're scanning – what's happening? I always ask my patients: What are you feeling and *where*? When we're babies, we're all body. Our brain and proprioception (our sense of our body in space) is all mapped through bodily receptors, signifiers which are entirely sensory. That's what we need to get back to – a form of simple functioning, where we tap into our most primitive organisation, and forget all the jumbled thinking, the chat, the bullshit; the stuff which inflames us and often makes us angry. Instead, we just need to be asking: What am I feeling? And why?

The 'Why' is your pocket therapist.

What am I feeling? 'It's 10am, my heart is racing. My stomach hurts.'

Why? 'My boss shouted at me and intimated I was a stupid woman who wasn't welcome here and isn't as good as my male co-worker who's younger than me and is basically non-verbal.'

And then a further 'Why?' Maybe the answer would go something like: 'It's painful for me to ask myself this more deeply, because it's reminding me that, even though I was told all the way through school that my hard work would assure me a way out of my unambitious town and also my undermining family, it seems I've hit the same obstacle further down this road. This time, in the form of an abusively undermining boss. What can I do?'

Stay and repair

In psychotherapy, 'stay and repair' is the name of the game with conflict of any type, including the type of internal conflict we feel when we really want to get out of a situation which feels unbearable to us. This is when tuning in to the specifics of our affect system is really helpful. What are you feeling *in your body*? Where are you feeling it? In your stomach? What type of sensation? The uncomfortable fluttering of adrenaline, a leaden ache of dread? A cold, falling sensation, as if every organ was dropping out of you?

Get used to categorising the sensations as familiar or not. If familiar, what do they remind you of? 'This is like when Dad said he'd take me to go shopping, but he never showed up to collect me ...' or 'This is like when I found out my friends had gone to a festival without me, as they told me I was too boring' or 'This is just like when my mum told me her cancer had come back.'

However large or small the feelings, start to pay attention and draw the threads together. When we know the type of response we're likely to have *in extremis*, we're better prepared and can also understand why we feel something so keenly, what our body is telling us that it's reminded of and warning us about. Being cognisant of the parallels helps us bring our thinking back online, even when we're under emotional pressure. Our brain might try to tell us that this situation is different, but our body knows another truth.

What we want to get ourselves adept at is the capacity to keep our thinking, our logical mind, online, whilst making the most of what our emotional apparatus is providing. This is the raw data we need in order to make the best informed, most superior decisions which optimise our power. When we know why our body's gone wild in its reaction, we can help to steady our thoughts. 'Don't worry – I know this feels like the time when the whole class started laughing at you. But that's not what's happening here. You're an adult now. You're safe.' Then you're free to use the original information, gathered more purely from your environment, without it being clouded by your projections.

Our 'affective equipment' – our body sensations, our emotions, our felt responses – really *are* the Geiger counter with which we read rooms. When people are in positions of lower power and status, they get good at this. It's a form of hypervigilance and most women are pretty adept at it, agile as we are at adapting around the moods and needs of others, ducking angry fathers' outbursts, dodging stronger brothers' swipes, working out how to slide away from this man without him killing us, wheeling around the underhand meanness of other girls. Let's use it now to our advantage. It really is a superpower, if we can harness it to work *with* us. We want to make use of it now to establish the safest, most effective way of staying in the room, instead of helping us to calculate the swiftest way out.

Now that you've worked out what you're feeling, you need to start expressing it cogently and in a way which prioritises best outcome. For you. Using 'I feel' statements is usually a pretty safe approach here. You'll be good at this, if you're regulated and tuning in to what those feelings actually consist of. You'll present something more certain and less equivocal, because you understand the solid data these readings are based on.

'*I feel* quite taken advantage of in this situation' … '*I feel* you haven't heard what I've said to you' … '*I feel* you prioritised what the men in the room were saying in that meeting, and didn't give me space to articulate my thoughts' … '*I feel* that my emotions and needs were not taken into account, when you decided that I would be the primary carer for my brother' … '*I feel* that you don't consider the thought that goes into making dinner every night of the week' … '*I feel* you just expect me to pick up the childcare shortfall in the school holidays and assume that my job will accommodate this. Which *I feel* is highly disrespectful and not based in any kind of reality where you take me and my profession seriously. This is not the brand of equality I signed up for'… and so on.

We then give the other person space to express their point: 'This is my mind on the situation – what's yours?' Remember, *keep breathing*, keep tuning in to your gut. Notice your reactions. Keep your mind open and curious. We have no idea how we're impacting the other person. They may find this type of straightforward, pure communication extremely confronting. There's something disarming about someone who can obey their basic responses and react to them in a simple, authentic way. In the best sense, it's quite childlike and guileless. And in a world where people have tangled themselves up in sophisticated knots to ensure that sexism is hidden away, someone openly and uncomplicatedly calling it out is powerful. So the recipient may be a little taken aback, which feels like an elegant reversal of all the multiple times we've been caught on the back foot and unable to respond.

Stay in the room

Whenever it was that it started, we women need to decide *here*'s where the buck stops. We need to put on the brakes and make the changes; we need to say no to *our* bodies and *our* minds being the soft tissue on which that legacy of exploitation finds another yielding surface. We need to say No, and we need to say it in the moment. However we do it. With humour. With playfulness. We need to use the resources centuries of oppression have afforded us, the skillset to rival any number of armies. We have the nouse, the 'emotional intelligence' (was there ever a more downgraded form of intelligence?). The controlling forces were too short-sighted to realise that it was exactly the qualities that spelt our 'weakness' which actually turn out to be our most chillingly effective weapons.

The other thing we need to remember is how urgent and critical it is that we stay to support each other. Women are incredible. We have the capacity (thanks in part to a shared history relegated to lowly status) for a deep relational richness, which we must now use to our best communal advantage. So many social structures are designed to pit us against each other – from social media to hair products, to not being allowed to overtly voice feelings of aggression and rage. When we struggle to tell each other about our angry feelings, we deprive ourselves of the chance to grow and evolve. We owe it to each other and ourselves to have the uncomfortable conversations, instead of walking away, ghosting each other or bitching behind backs.

To this end, I urge women to always try and 'stay in the room'. Whilst all of our reflexes are screaming Get Out, we need to fight the fear and resist the urge to crawl into bed and hide under the duvet, lamenting What's The Point? The point is, *you got yourself here*. You've got what it takes to stay. Dig deep, thank your brilliantly attuned affect system for telling you that you prefer to scarper from that family member who makes you feel so small. And now, reach beyond that alarm to locate your desire.

This also applies to our professional lives. Remind yourself that this job has always been your goal. It's what every late-night cramming session was for. And even if it's not about the job itself, even if it's more about having had enough of being diminished and having choices taken away, you deserve those choices. Possibly more than the younger man now sitting in the position above you. Fight for yourself, as you would encourage your friend to, or your little sister, or your daughter. Do it for Older Woman you. Do it because, even if you only want it sometimes, that guy wanted it less and has no fighting to do.

Book in the space with your boss. Go formal. Give no wiggle room. If you're prepared, you're protected. Do your homework.

What do you want to say? Do you have evidence? Evidence is our absolute ally. Save it all. Take notes, make a diary, make a log. Bring it all. Do you want to take someone in for moral support? A trusted colleague? Before you go in, write exactly what you want to say. And if you're too afraid to do anything else, just read it out. Say you'll forward your points to them after the meeting. Sexism is operating covertly, and we need to flush it out at every opportunity. No more of our bodies adapting and getting better at absorbing all of the hits. We've had enough. Get it in writing.

This is the road to assertiveness. This is the road to standing our ground. When we say: I'm not a child who has no choice but to comply. I'm now an adult, who sees where that feeling comes from and decides to do things differently.

We're not repressing the feeling, we're acknowledging it. And responding to something else. This is no longer our cue to leave. No more shuffling off after having babies and battling menopause. That ends here. We stay in the room, metaphorically speaking: we override the urge to flee, no matter how uncomfortable and unfamiliar this feels. And we demand better. Something *is* wrong, but the solution *isn't* to run away. And if you're not happy with the apology, or the pay-off, you stay longer. We think our body can't take any more of it, but leaving just means we're left bearing the wound.

We stay and fight, and we throw our anger back in. Use your anger when you feel there's no fight left. Wear a wide smile, because you feel so happy to have the opportunity to *not* be carrying it with you. Ask Mara, who would say her work caused her cancer. Ask Didi, who would say the only way of coping with the rage she felt towards her vile father was by numbing herself internally with blankets of food, forming a layer to protect herself from the inside. Or Tamara, who got written off with PND.

The first key part of feeling released from our repressed rage is truly being able to tune in to our feelings. The second part is being able to express them clearly. Let's think in more detail about how this can best be achieved.

Give Yourself a Vocabulary

As women, we simply don't have a suitable vocabulary with which to express feelings of anger. We need to go back to the years where we should have been taught it – essentially, the primitive years of infancy, where language is being laid down and our brains are programming themselves around symbols and codes. At some primary schools now, children are encouraged to check in daily with their feelings, using a colour chart. They're supported to elaborate on the colour they choose for their mood that day and to think about what's made them feel that way. In short, they're not told what they're *supposed* to feel, they're given room to tap in and explore what they *actually* feel. Revolutionary. Life-changing. And so simple.

Ideally, our parents would have given us this toolkit. That whole 'use your words' idea should really be – 'Feel your feelings!' And then 'Let's find the words together for those feelings!' With those loving, tuned-in parents, we'd have started to build an internal map of our emotions and what they're telling us, and why they're telling us what they're telling us. Instead, for most of us, feelings have to knock extremely loudly on the door to our consciousness before we begin to pay any attention or take them seriously. People turn up for therapy when things have reached a disastrous stage. They're on their knees or their minds have completely snapped. They'll go for a fast fix of a few months' treatment and then, often, off they'll go again, without taking seriously any of the processes which have resulted in them coming here in the first place.

These habits of not listening, and of allowing other people to disregard our emotions, took years of wiring to establish. It's going to take time and some commitment to get ourselves unravelled, which, you might argue, could be seen as a source of anger in its own right. Why should we be left with the bill that our parents, who decided to put us on this planet, incurred on our behalf? Indeed so. But where does this end? How did it begin? With the shit parenting they had, with the Second World War (which definitely fucked up at least a generation), with the 'Enlightenment'?!

If you find it difficult to label your feelings – especially your angry ones – with accuracy (as many of us do, who haven't benefitted from modern education techniques or thoughtful parenting) start with the colour method yourself. You could then move on to numbers.

For example: 'I'm feeling Red 4/5 and Blue 1/5.'

Try finding simple words to describe this: 'I'm more angry than sad.'

Think more deeply: 'I'm really frustrated, I feel disrespected, patronised.'

Why? 'Because of how I'm being treated in my team.'

Where are you feeling that? 'The anger is in my stomach, the sadness is in my chest and throat.'

Is the feeling familiar? Does it remind you of other times in your life? Is it so resonant *because* it's historic?

As I say, when we're feeling overwhelmed by a sensation, it's extremely helpful to label it and to separate past from present. You're an Adult Woman now. Not a hostage to an earlier, more helpless life stage.

Use Anger Better

So, you've stayed in the room. Having identified some of the feelings you're flooded by, it might be good to discharge some of the excess energy they've brought along, whether you're calling it anger or anxiety. This will help you reregulate. Go and do star jumps in the loo, punch a cushion, ball a jumper up into your mouth and scream, or yell into a pillow ... Whatever it is, wherever you are, don't be thinking about how to 'manage your anxiety' anymore – dare yourself to interpret this energy as rage, even if it doesn't immediately present as that, and get shot of some of the heat of it. Think of yourself as a racehorse, bred for incredible application of targeted energy. When racehorses are raring to go, they sweat and foam and can't keep still – you can see the adrenaline coursing through their raised capillaries. This is how we need to think of ourselves. We're *trained* for this. All of the battening down and gagging and dismissal, all of the late nights cramming because your confidence would never let you just breeze into an exam. That roar which was repressed the first time men stared at you in your new hot pants. '*They're not for you!*' You wanted to scream. 'I bought them for me! With my pocket money!' That 13-year-old you is still inside you. We're doing this *for her*. For that little girl who didn't know what was going on and certainly didn't have the resources to do anything about it. She was a good girl and she said sorry to those men, who blocked her path and continued to stare. But she was there, biding her time, gaining in power, gaining in knowledge. Big knowledge, big thoughts. Big capacities. And we're going to unleash them now.

Deep breaths. Centre yourself. There are a hundred fast hacks for this online: alternate nostril breathing, pressure points, visualisations. Get things settled and stable. Allow your thinking to come back online. Plan what you want to say, as simply as possible, using your 'I' statements. And *get back in that room*.

Build Team Woman

Let's create a movement. If we can get better at vocalising the negative emotions we have for each other, and not walling them up and releasing them as well-timed put-downs or backstabbing, then the sense is that we're part of a team, a supportive army which has our back and knows the game plan. If not, we're actually left doing the work of the patriarchy. Because of how projection works, that means we're really running *ourselves* down.

Again, we're attempting to undo generations of wiring here, across all levels – from the way others relate to us, to how we relate to each other. When we know that our women have our back, it's much easier to stand our ground. Thus fortified, stay in the room. Stay and play. Get back in and fight. If your voice trembles, it's probably worth saying. Use your anger to fuel your determination. Get on and do what you need to do – don't be floored by the emotion of it. Separate the emotions from the thoughts; separate one feeling from the other. Tease out what's excess. Ditch that. Take the important bit and *get back in there*.

The reason I keep repeating the need to 'get back in' is because we naturally find it so hard to stand our ground when it's happening, and to say it as it arises. Over time, this gets easier. The more adept we get at hearing our feelings and taking them seriously, the less we feel frightened and floored by them. Remember, other people don't *make* us feel anything. Two people will have two very different responses to the same event. What's traumatic for one woman isn't universally so. This means that it really is our own historic apparatus which hijacks us, and which we need to get more of a handle on, in order to use emotion to our advantage, not be squashed by it.

A historic strategy for keeping ourselves safe when communicating with other women is self-diminishment – when we self-deprecate or say something 'wasn't that hard', or that something about us 'isn't great'. Though another woman may be offering us a well-intentioned compliment, we're actually doing something which *feels* self-protective by handing it back. We're trying to ward off envious attack. So often, what women fear from each other is the disguised insult or the complex 'I want to be you, but also I hate you' sentiment. Thus, keeping ourselves closed to the offering feels like a good idea in the moment. It feels prudent. In fact, though, we're handing over our power. Self-abasement can also feel like rejection to the other person offering us a genuine gift – they've bothered to give you something that may have cost them – and you throw it aside. In throwing away the offering, we deprive *her* of her power. That energy floats into the ether like so much steam or smoke, a by-product of a reaction which leaves us burnt out, with nothing to show for the exchange.

We need to reclaim that energy – if another woman gives you something, accept it with grace and gratitude. Make her feel that her opinion's worthwhile and allow the warm reaction that can kindle something between people to establish itself. You'll both walk away with a spring in your step instead of shuffling off, unsure whether you dodged some sort of a bullet, and her feeling as if you threw one at her. Paranoia and suspicion are the enemy here; both ways of ultimately causing ourselves harm – which is ironic when those feelings are sold as tools of self-protection. This isn't how our emotional apparatus should be used. We need to retrain it to identify the real attack. Yes, that may feel larger and more nebulous and lifelong – and where the hell do you begin? It's much easier to side-step a perceived slight from a woman at work or in the playground than to try taking down the patriarchy brick by brick. What we don't realise when we focus it on other women, and see the attacks as emanating *from* them, is that we actually reinforce the fortress of misogyny in the process.

Don't be Afraid of Feeling

Fundamentally, we need to ask ourselves, what's wrong with strong emotion? There are trigger warnings everywhere now, and it seems we'd rather label ourselves as having some sort of *hard*wiring disorder, than look at why certain emotions and situations *feel* so unbearable for us. We've flipped from a time in which we mustn't show feeling because it's somehow unseemly and uncouth, to a time when we mustn't show feeling because it upsets us and those around us too much. In one of the first processing group sessions I held in order to give women a space to feel and talk about their anger, someone approached me afterwards and said that I should have warned people we would talk about feelings. I reminded her that the whole purpose of the group had been arranged around this particular feeling. Yes, *but what if someone had felt something too much?* I said, I'm a therapist, there's no such thing as too much feeling. It's what I do. I've done it with violent offenders. I've done it with extremely disturbed psychotic patients. Feelings don't frighten me. And yet, her risk aversion said it all. This is the conditioning: women are taught to be afraid of expressing their stronger, negative feelings, and being around other people when *they* do. It's possibly evolutionary, when you think about it. We're scared we'll be killed if we push it or assert a need, so better keep the peace.

It seems as if, nowadays, we're happier giving ourselves a label based around our organic circuitry, rather than focusing on our internal universe of feeling and discovering what it has to tell us. The messages from our feelings are initially quite intimidating, so maybe it's easier to take ourselves *out of the room* and claim that our neurological label (whether that's our social anxiety or attachment style) makes it difficult for us to be in there, surrounded by all of that emotion. But humans are great at feelings! We're the mammals that use them in the most creative, sophisticated ways. We combine them with our knowledge of death and existence to work out how to apply them to our advantage. If, as women especially, we deny them, cut them off and distance ourselves from their messages ever further, we lose the very thing that offers us power. The goods we're already carrying, which years in the wilderness have strengthened.

GET IT ALL OUT

Let's start feeling it. Let's feel it all. And, as an extension to that pledge: let's stop apologising for saying what we feel. We're frightened about hurting others with our feelings. It's almost as if society at some point clocked our superpower – *that we're emotionally exceptional* – and hastily sought to quash this with messages of 'being kind' and 'if you can't say anything nice' and 'now you're showing off'. As women, we're used to being trapped inside other people's projections and demands. From our earliest family attachments, we're conditioned to react and respond to cues to perform along certain lines of expectation. Awareness of this allows us options. If we can identify the anger that conditioning incites in us, we can evolve responses which are more beneficial to us. We can also experiment with taking up the opposing position whereby we dare to invert the expectations we've internalised, and just see what happens if we allow the other person to feel *our* emotion for a change.

It's of note that, these days, corporate buzz-speak clusters around 'using vulnerability' in decision-making. This is funny, when you consider that, pretty recently, it used to be the rather more masculine-sounding 'resilience' that was de rigueur in the business world. 'Management' has suddenly cottoned on that the superskill of those women now permitted a seat at the table was the self-same valueless 'emotional intelligence' so previously minimised. *Thank you ladies!* We'll take the spoils you're offering, and rebrand them as if we dreamt them up. 'Feminine weakness' becomes 'vulnerability', and is charming and valuable in a man. *Thanks for the great ideas, lady.* Now get lost and let me promote my friend, who's written about using their EQ on their application (and who I also went to school with).

Our 'emotional intelligence' makes us sensitive to other

people's feelings, which means we're likely to be cautious about hurting people with our own articulated feelings. We're taught that we need to be careful with what we say, and very careful with how we express ourselves. This means we're left with the impression that we can make people feel things. Actually, we generally can't. OK, perhaps you can if you go all out to be mean to someone, targeting their weak spots and insecurities. Then, yuck, what sort of a person are you? What we're talking about here is the reality that, as a woman, you're probably far more likely to be worrying about telling someone how *you* feel and worrying that *you* must be the one in the wrong, that your very thoughts and feelings are the wrong things. We're so busy feeling wrong and bad that we're held back from expressing a lot of other potential feelings – including anger – which is another well-trodden way in which society really does a number on us. The very fabric on which every institution and idea is built is predicated on the idea of men's superiority and power. We're born into a landscape which inhibits our own feelings of rightness and self-confidence. We must dare to allow ourselves to be the correct ones; the ones who aren't fundamentally just 'wrong'.

Have Straightforward Conversations

Imagine how tall we'd allow ourselves to walk if the assumption was that we were *right*, that people loved us for who we were at a deep and simple level; if we knew our ideas and feelings would be met with applause and celebration. In that spirit of confidence, if we then discovered that something we'd said or done had in fact had a negative impact on someone, it might feel easier to suggest a conversation requiring both parties to take stock. We'd do it from a place not of anguish and our stomach having dropped out, but from somewhere stable and calm.

Finding our neutral helps us get better at having honest, straightforward conversations about feeling. It allows us to go in with a more observational: 'When you said this to me, I found myself feeling … I wonder if we could have a chat about that together? Maybe it's something I need to look at in myself, but I also felt you should know that it had an impact.' Imagine that level of maturity amongst adults … Because, actually, even if someone says the dreaded and appalling words, 'You hurt me!', we haven't actually inserted a particular feeling wholesale under their skin. Something happens *in them* which completes the reaction, like two chemicals combining. We relate to others, or their behaviours, in a way which is deeply informed by past experiences and people. We may not have a conscious knowledge of who or what that is, but our cells remember.

Although we're responsible for the words we use, we can't ever be held fully accountable for the specific impact they have on the other person. We can't control that. We might think we're 'making' someone feel loved and cherished and wind up with them feeling stifled or patronised. We just can't completely predict the outcome or the precise reaction that someone will have to our behaviour. Even if we're being good and nice and polite, we might be triggering buried memories of some backstabbing girl at school. They don't remember this consciously: they just know they don't like you. There are some things we simply can't control.

By implication, if the person standing opposite us has a particularly difficult reaction to something we've expressed about our own feelings, *they* have the opportunity to look at that in themselves. Imagine the *liberation* of expecting the person who's reacted negatively to 'do the work' on their own response instead of us feeling mortified and hastily falling on our swords. Our fear of upsetting typically means we avoid the expression of more frank or impassioned emotions. We *shrink*.

Ultimately, the solution to keeping anger away in the long term is Ordinary Conversation. Between everyone, men and women. We all need to talk more: about uncomfortable truths and dilemmas and apparent obstacles. From monthly periods to our personal safety when walking late at night, to the pay gap. To how boys and men can start taking on the emotional load, and sharing in our experiences more. *When* we can talk frankly and honestly about our vulnerabilities and fears, about our confusion and anger, and *when* we can invite men equally and non-defensively into the discussion alongside us, perhaps we won't be forced to suffer in such violent, internalised ways.

Stop Labelling

When we see other women as 'out to get us', when we label other women, we play into the constructs of patriarchy. When we label ourselves, we do the same thing. Diagnosing ourselves with all manner of health disorders – from dizzy spells to depression – we cancel ourselves out *for them*. The classic inventories used in primary healthcare settings corroborate that it's apparently easier for medicine to ask whether a woman is disordered, rather than angry.

We're missing a valuable opportunity to intercept women's care at a level which costs little, but which may ultimately get them more targeted help. If we're being honest, we know that the store of kinetic energy from unspent rage trapped inside of us would have us swear, hurl ourselves around, smear excrement across the walls of powerful and inhibiting institutions, and vomit our guts and bile over every person who's ever stared, made comments, denigrated us, minimised us, told us to be ladylike, calm down or girls don't do …We know that.

A kick-boxing class and ten sessions of talking therapy with a psychodynamic counsellor, trained to quickly get their hands dirty in the transference of past and present relationships, may save a lifetime's bafflement, expensive tests and procedures yielding inconclusive results (or minimal success with anti-depressants). Even six sessions of group therapy for 'angry women' (by which I mean all women) could efficiently provide safe, non-judgemental spaces for us to express our neatly tucked-away rage. I dream of an NHS plate-smashing room, underwater screaming classes at the municipal pool, mass hollering into wipe-clean cushions … We need to create a language, and readily available channels, for talking in an ordinary way about everyday feelings of injustice, rage, oppression and regret – rather than just giving them labels.

In therapy, I want patients to take an active role in their treatment. We think together about how to continue the work of the session outside. 'Observations' ('journals', if you will) are kept, events are recorded, experimental conversations are had and reported back on. As your pocket therapist, I can encourage you to become *your own* therapist, just as I encourage my patients. I hope some of these ideas strengthen you and become a bit of an inner voice, like a sensible parent advising what you probably already know you should do, but tend to forget. As I said, I call this an 'internal scaffold': to listen carefully to your body, to trust your body and to trust your instinct. To know you're not wrong, and that actually other people can be the wrong ones. And to behave according to these new rules. The ones you should have had all along. The basics.

What we can do

- Learn to regulate our bodies.
- Regularly scan our feelings.
- Remember, a healthy brain is one which moves regularly through diverse feeling states.
- Allow a clear channel of communication. Learn to say what you feel. In the moment.
- Talk about everything in families, schools and workplace – no topic barred, from periods to domestic violence.
- Stop separating boys and girls, in what we expect of them, and in more practical ways.
- Bring boys into the conversation from before they can speak.
- Ask those boys, and keep asking as they become men, What can we do about this? How can we discuss our envious, resentful feelings before they calcify into anger?
- Together, learn to frame the question, 'Can we Have It All?' I suspect we can.

Final Note: What Now?

IN WRITING ABOUT the feelings that women bring me, I thought it would be possible to be objective and measured in tone, my voice more powerful for its distance and passive positioning. The data collection technique of psychotherapy would confidently furnish me with evidence, just as it furnishes and informs me in the consulting room. Therapy is a natural process, occurring within the real world, as opposed to laboratory settings, and, as such, allows me a window into how humans naturally operate and the behaviours exhibited outside of the consulting room.

However, as I moved objectively through the case studies, logging examples of everyday micro- and macro-acts of brazen, socially legitimised violations of women's well-being by employers, medical professionals, partners and parents, I grew increasingly unable to moderate my own feelings of anger. I couldn't remain the 'researcher'. I noticed my physiology respond in ways which mirrored those of my patients. These women's experiences resonate with my own, as well as those of my friends and female relatives, and my body won't let me forget that. In allowing them to reverberate in me, these feelings of anger grow more strident and authoritative. Understanding dawns on me. We're in a new era of female shutdown. Misogynistic structures find new ways to get around the templates we've put in place to protect us.

What I've realised is that, at a certain point, these symptoms go beyond the privacy of the individual. When this many women describe the same set of 'symptoms', the same pattern of causes, we should sit up and take notice. As professionals, we need to admit that something has still not been addressed at a psychosocial level. That, in fact, something about the myth that it *has* been – that we're now emancipated – precludes our argument and further silences us. The lie acts against us. And, worse still, we're doing it to ourselves. We're participants in our own destruction. It's an own-goal.

As I moved through my writing, competing feelings arrived in me. If this really is the beginning of a new wave of feminism, was I endangering myself to wed myself to it? It's hardly clinically neutral, after all. However, I think the wider sense of female shutdown was at play here as well – a kind of frightened, wired-in misogyny gagged me, too. I worried about being cancelled, about ruffling feathers, about upsetting medic colleagues who might feel I was criticising their dedication and pouring scorn on their careworn and struggling services. We're suddenly living in a much less predictable world, which feels more unsafe. We really haven't had our privileges for very long. And it's always the last ones in, those of us grudgingly granted a token seat at the table, who'll be the most disposable when things get tougher. Take heed women. We'll always be witches to some. Witches or whores.

And the more they desire us, the more their hatred grows. The more they envy our power, the more they'll seek to destroy us. I've now seen how hard it is to keep the torch lit, to keep banging the drum when many people want to cover their ears. Men who are fearful and conflicted. Women who don't want their husbands to see them as angry or unattractive, and seek to flatter male egos as a more familiar way of keeping themselves protected. To turn to face the wall is to fast-forward our own fate. As the world burns and populations resort to ever more desperate means to survive, the oppressed will be the first to fall, the first to face sacrifice.

This is a systemic misogyny, in which men are also victims. Men themselves are increasingly coming forward for psychotherapy and, based on my work with them, I see how they too are caught within a system in which roles are still so crudely and stereotypically drawn. Men can also seem frozen, uncertain of how to behave – what he can say, what he can ask for, how to express his needs in a world which seeks to polarise and divide the sexes. Men feel stymied, impotent and misunderstood. Men and women are backed into corners, afraid of each other.

Moving into the future, using an unequivocal lexicon is necessary in order to call out passive abuses and redistribute power. Terms like microaggression, financial abuse, gaslighting, hazing and gagging are all useful ways of shining light on these processes. We must ensure that these terms don't get misappropriated and misused in ways which devalue their meaning. Communication has to be the way to find connection through this landscape. We need clear language expressing clear mechanisms which we're all getting better at identifying. We need to feel more confident in speaking honestly with each other from the earliest age, in order to build a shared language capable of liberating us from these dead-end positions.

I sometimes wonder if the way we talk about 'women's issues' is part of the reality perpetuating them. If you introduced a rallying speech with:

'Half of the current global population is afraid to walk the streets of their town when night falls …'

Or: 'Addressing the global 75 per cent who are carers …'

Or: '49.74 per cent of the global population is afraid to sit on a white sofa …'

Or: '64 million jobs were lost due to the COVID-19 pandemic! Translating to $800 billion dollars' worth of income!'

… Then more would happen.

By categorising these realities as 'women's issues', we allow ourselves to become erased, patronised and denigrated. Our stock is frozen low.

But there's also a problem with calling us all, men and women alike, 'the people'. We do have different needs as women. But men can learn to listen better. We can learn to tell them better. These are woman's issues, but they affect us all. Instead of shutting down on these experiences and giving up on change, we could all just talk about them more.

A fear of saying the wrong thing means men shy away from such conversations. Their trademark silence is perceived as 'strong', but maybe it's actually frightened and confused. We, as women, can decide to plough forward anyway, starting with an ordinary approach to talking about our bodies and bodily experiences. Our daughters ditching the shame connected with so many aspects of their lives provides confidence and frees up their energy. That confident energy keeps the conversation fresh and alive. We're talking about an adapted feminism for where we are now, for the world we live in now, where problems are best tackled together.

With a more straightforward attitude to our bodies and discussion of our embodied experience, we can more easily ask for the things we need in life – from our families, partners and healthcare providers, to employers and eventually politicians. Women aren't just small men or men with extra bits stuck onto our bodies. We're different to men. And, for too long now, we've been trying to behave as if we're the same, with the same privileges and freedoms. Let's stop pretending, let's be more realistic. Different is just as good. We don't need to be afraid of it or diminish that difference. We can feel more congruent with ourselves and those around us if we stop pretending and own this difference. We can be realistic about hormonal events and the language of our bodies, without shame. From this frank and open place, we can ask for the things we really need, and recognise when those things aren't provided. We don't need to be driven to such angry and unwell places before we start to understand what we're missing.

On a wider note, perhaps we as a society have got our priorities wrong. The more we earn and expect to earn, the more we push up our own prices. We're all contributing, not only to economic inflation, but to the inflation of our mental health problems. Perhaps it isn't possible to raise psychologically healthy, balanced young people when we expect the impossible of ourselves. We aren't modelling something moderate and 'good enough', in the words of the paediatrician-psychoanalyst Donald Winnicott. We're instead creating a template where dissatisfaction and envy are the name of the game, and men and women are pitted against each other in a race to the psychological bottom.

Women are, naturally, the current losers. But I don't think men are far behind. Typically, men land their anxiety or insecurity on women as rage, inducing fearful shutdown and resigned acquiescence in her. The use of wife as therapist fundamentally does her harm. Men are also victims of this old-fashioned system. I know, from my personal and professional experience, that men can feel as trapped and undignified by the process and structures of patriarchy as women. They wouldn't choose for things to shake down this way. But they mustn't come and dump that on us. We need more than that, in the face of a social system keeping these problems very much alive in increasingly devious and outrageous ways. By learning to talk from the earliest ages about our differences and similarities, we can work together to give ourselves what we need. Perhaps all genders trying to conform to traditional ideas of 'masculinity' as king enslaves us all to a system which is basically just how capitalism best entraps us. Is this what we *really* want?

Revolution

As the case studies in each chapter demonstrate, there *is* another way – another way of organising our health, our lifestyles and our relationships. You've joined me on a journey from cradle to grave. Together, we've surveyed the landscape into which we arrive, and currently struggle to live within. A landscape which renders our screams silent and which ultimately often kills us off. We've learnt how crucial it is to identify the rage and that we must process or discharge it. Our body has been the container for all of this feeling, and now we need to use it properly – as a tool of recovery and empowerment, rather than an object which endangers and co-opts us. Anger as a pro-social emotion. Anger as fuel.

As we've seen, a brain in pain causes a cascade of inflammatory signalling, alerting the body to a high-risk internal situation. Everything is braced, reactions will be heightened. The system is under attack and we respond accordingly.

In spite of the substantial progress made in the field of mental health across the last 40 years, from knowledge around the impact of a human's environment to epigenetics to genomics, to these more recent revelations around inflammation, the key cause of major mood disorders has eluded us. As have the reasons for the dominant rates of major depression in women. It's as if the primitive brain has a limited range of responses to injury, and anxiety and depression is the ultimate common route, accessible by numerous pathways. What we're realising is that our brains hurting in this pervasive, chronic and underground way can *cause* our bodies to hurt. This book, by tracing a contemporary journey from a woman's babyhood to her death, has attempted to shed light on the causes of our suffering. And what we can do to reverse these catastrophic effects.

Like A Girl

She drives just like a girl you know
She throws just like one too
She fights just like a girl as well
She's just no match for you

She also runs just like a girl
And there's the way she plays
But when they say 'just like a girl'
I think they mean to say

Worse
And somehow less
Somehow slower, somehow weaker
They think that if she's 'like a girl'
They'll easily defeat her

But girls will go to battle
When they already are bleeding
And girls are great at throwing themselves
Upwards through glass ceilings

Girls are busy navigating progress,
Driving change
And girls are busy winning
Whilst you criticise their game

FINAL NOTE: WHAT NOW?

So tell her that she's 'like a girl' –
She may just prove you right
She may out-play, out-last you,
Win the race and win the fight

'Cause she's a driving force
Fighting for her place in this world
And if you try to talk her down
She'll rise up

Like a girl

By Becky Hemsley

Acknowledgements

HOW COULD I not write this book? And how would it have been possible, without the unfailing support and championship of my keystones? Thanks go to:

My remarkable agent and trusted sage, Elly James. My incredible editor Michelle Signore, who instantly saw what I saw, and how urgent it was that everyone else see it. To my copy editor, Julia Kellaway, for her delicacy and intellectual rigour. And to Madiya Altaf, Matt Phillips, Eleanor Stammeijer, Tamara Douthwaite, Charlotte Brown and everyone at Bonnier. Your work on my behalf has bowled me over.

Professor Jennifer Graham-Engeland, my mentor and now friend. Sabine Nollau, my clinical supervisor and so much more. To Anouchka Grose, my stable ground and calm brain. To Linda Harakis, for getting me to this point.

The WAM community and our loyal listeners. You make it all worthwhile.

Salima. If I don't *literally* hear your voice in my ear, I hear your voice in my ear. And what would I be without it?

Thanks, too, to: Andie, my pillar and my heart; Scout, spokesperson for the next generation; Jenny B, my go-to and oracle in everything; Tammy, for giving up her time and precious brain; Mel, without whom it's *all* impossible; Ekow, who showed me how to channel my rage; Helen R, for early steering; Hannah, my cousin and finest Anger Ambassador; Tamsin, for your constancy and deep camaraderie; Katy, equally driven, for *getting it*; Sarah-Lou, who got the book ball rolling; Giles, for your insight and eternal largesse; Maria, for your generosity and emphasis of how critical this was; Fran, for hearing me out in the early days and making this feel possible; Olly, natural-born writer and lifelong advocate; Lulu, for bringing that academic perspective and wider, wiser view; Frog, for understanding *why*. My new friend Stacey, for your openheartedness. Charlotte and Jamie, for your backing and belief; Juliet, movie star and sister in the cause; Julie B, for fondant fancies and cheerleading; Jonathan and Laura, for your journalistic eye.

To Andrea, Antonella, Judith, Julie, Mags, Caro, Lynn, Tara: always on my side; Shappi, for your support from the get-go; Soraya, a figurehead in a stormy sea; Tilly, for showing me what Instagram was, as we propped up our corner; Jane, for launching us into orbit; Ania and Kordian, who sustained me from afar; Office Party – Abby, Jenny P, Karen: my Life Raft and lungs; Ify, for your straightforward generosity; the Weymouth Girls, for putting up with me.

To my deeply feminist family, who taught me how to wire plugs, change tyres and ask 'Why?' (and for encouraging the gastrointestinal surgery on my dolls).

To Sally, for whom I learnt how to fight.

To Simon. The best of men, the truest team-mate.

To my beautiful boys, the hope of a brighter tomorrow.

Endnotes

Introduction

Page 3 Women are twice as likely as men to suffer depression
Anxiety and Depression Association of America (n.d.). Women and depression.
Retrieved from https://adaa.org/find-help-for/women/depression.

Page 3 Women are ... three times more likely to experience migraines
Walter, K. (2022). What is migraine? *JAMA, 327*(1), 93.

Page 3 Women are ... four times more likely to be diagnosed with autoimmune disease
Kronzer, V. L., Bridges Jr, S. L., & Davis III, J. M. (2021). Why women have more autoimmune diseases than men: An evolutionary perspective. *Evolutionary Applications, 14*(3), 629–33.

Page 3 There seems to have been a global pivot away from sexual parity after agricultural economies began to dominate, as we shifted to a more sedentary way of life.
Lockard, C. A. (2014). *Societies, Networks, and Transitions: A Global History.* Cengage Learning, 88–9.

Page 3 Darwin himself had some choice views on sex differences and, indeed, promoted the finding that women were inferior in body and mind.
Darwin, C. (1896). *The Descent of Man and Selection in Relation to Sex.* D. Appleton and Company.

Bergman, G. (2002). The history of the human female inferiority ideas in evolutionary biology. *Rivista di biologia*, *95*(3), 379–412.

Page 3 There have been countless opportunities to address these issues, since the word 'sexism' was immortalised by the US feminist Caroline Bird Mahoney more than half a century ago in her speech, 'On Being Born Female'.
City News Publishing Company (1969). *Vital Speeches of the Day 1968–1969*, *35*(3), 90.

Page 5 A *patriarchal* world; a world where history, geography, privilege and structure have been dominated by men.
Hunnicutt, G. (2009). Varieties of patriarchy and violence against women: Resurrecting 'patriarchy' as a theoretical tool. *Violence Against Women*, *15*(5), 553–73.

Chapter One: You're Being Gaslit

Page 12 Indeed, recent data from the campaign Pregnant Then Screwed found that 52 per cent of women face discrimination during their pregnancy, maternity leave or on return to work.
Pregnant Then Screwed (19 Jul. 2023). 1 in 61 pregnant women say their boss insinuated they should have an abortion. Retrieved from https://pregnantthenscrewed.com/1-in-61-pregnant-women-say-their-boss-insinuated-they-should-have-an-abortion/#:~:text=A%20new%20study%20from%20Pregnant,a%20negative%20or%20discriminatory%20experience.

Chapter Two: What Anger Does to Our Bodies

Page 15 When there's a disparity between our expectation and reality, between what we were envisaging as a 'reward' and that being somehow thwarted, our amygdala (the brain region chiefly concerned with emotional processes) is alerted and feelings of anger flow.
Blair, R. J. R. (2012). Considering anger from a cognitive neuroscience perspective. *Wiley Interdisciplinary Reviews: Cognitive Science*, *3*(1), 65–74.

Page 16 Psychologists Stanley Schachter and Jerome Singer were key players in helping to illustrate the extent to which the *interpretation* of our emotions is key to our experience.
Schachter, S., & Singer, J. (1962). Cognitive, social, and physiological determinants of emotional state. *Psychological Review*, *69*(5), 379.

ENDNOTES

Page 17 Numerous meta-analyses find that the levels of those same acute-phase proteins and pro-inflammatory cytokines are elevated in patients with major depression.

Nemeroff, C. B. (2020). The state of our understanding of the pathophysiology and optimal treatment of depression: Glass half full or half empty? *American Journal of Psychiatry, 177*(8), 671–85.

Page 17 Let's consider the ordinary role of inflammation. It occurs when chemical mediators produced by the body's white blood cells enter the bloodstream and tissues.

Chen, L., Deng, H., Cui, H., Fang, J., Zuo, Z., Deng, J., ... & Zhao, L. (2018). Inflammatory responses and inflammation-associated diseases in organs. *Oncotarget, 9*(6), 7204–18.

Page 17 Damaged tissue sends its own chemical signals, to which white blood cells respond by releasing compounds prompting cellular division and tissue regrowth.

Punchard, N. A., Whelan, C. J., & Adcock, I. (2004). *The Journal of Inflammation, 1*, 1.

Page 17 In autoimmune diseases like arthritis, the immune system triggers inflammation unnecessarily, causing damage as it fights regular tissues as if they are infected or diseased.

Tanaka, Y. (2020). Rheumatoid arthritis. *Journal of Inflammation and Regeneration, 40*, 20.

Page 17 But longer-term elevations in inflammation have also been linked to the experience of chronic feelings of anger.

Castle, R., Bushell, W. J., Mills, P. J., Williams, M. A., Chopra, D., Rindfleisch, J. A. (12 Oct. 2021). Global Correlations Between Chronic Inflammation and Violent Incidents: Potential Behavioral Consequences of Inflammatory Illnesses Across Socio-Demographic Levels. *International Journal of General Medicine.* 14:6677-6691. doi: 10.2147/IJGM.S324367. PMID: 34675629; PMCID: PMC8520436.

Page 17 Over time, increased levels of inflammation can impact our cell DNA, and have been linked to diseases like diabetes and cancer, and even to obesity.

Coussens, L. M., Werb, Z. (2022). Inflammation and cancer. *Nature.* Dec. 19-26; 420(6917):860-7. doi: 10.1038/nature01322. PMID: 12490959; PMCID: PMC2803035.

Page 17 The bidirectional relationship of depression with autoimmune disease is firmly established, meaning that people with these diseases – from multiple sclerosis (MS) and autoimmune thyroiditis to IBS – are also likely to report major depression.
Euesden, J., Danese, A., Lewis, C. M., & Maughan, B. (2017). A bidirectional relationship between depression and the autoimmune disorders – New perspectives from the National Child Development Study. *PloS One, 12*(3), e0173015.

Coussens, L. M., & Werb, Z. (2002). Inflammation and cancer. *Nature, 420*(6917), 860–7.

Page 18 Both states of mind also seem to co-occur with inflammation, and repressed anger can function in part as a predisposing factor. Interestingly for us, the impact of early life trauma on inflammation is observed in patients with major depression.
Perozzo, P., Savi, L., Castelli, L., Valfrè, W., Lo Giudice, R., Gentile, S., ... & Pinessi, L. (2005). Anger and emotional distress in patients with migraine and tension–type headache. *The Journal of Headache and Pain, 6*, 392–9.

Page 18 Many researchers argue for the wealth of clinical and pre-clinical evidence that negative childhood events result in an ongoing elevation of pro-inflammatory cytokine secretion.
Grosse, L., Ambrée, O., Jörgens, S., Jawahar, M. C., Singhal, G., Stacey, D., ... & Baune, B. T. (2016). Cytokine levels in major depression are related to childhood trauma but not to recent stressors. *Psychoneuroendocrinology, 73*, 24–31.

Page 19 Surface electromyography (which measures muscle response) indicates recruitment of muscles across our upper arms and shoulders in tandem with the experience of angry emotion.
Huis in't Veld, E. M. J., Van Boxtel, G. J., & de Gelder, B. (2014). The Body Action Coding System I: Muscle activations during the perception and expression of emotion. *Social Neuroscience, 9*(3), 249–64.

Page 19 Studies have zoned in on the association between migraine and problems with the expression of anger, but more on that later.
Shaygan, M., Saranjam, E., Faraghi, A., & Mohebbi, Z. (2022). Migraine headaches: The predictive role of anger and emotional intelligence. *International Journal of Community Based Nursing and Midwifery, 10*(1), 74–83.

ENDNOTES

Page 19 All in, remaining in sustained states of suppressed anger can increase the likelihood of stroke, Type 2 diabetes, cardiovascular diseases and heart attacks.

Staicu, M. L., & Cuțov, M. (2010). Anger and health risk behaviors. *Journal of Medicine and Life*, *3*(4), 372–5.

Page 20 As we're beginning to learn, elevated inflammation readings are physically destructive. In this case, they can increase our risk of pulmonary disease.

Lehrer, P. (2006). Anger, stress, dysregulation produces wear and tear on the lung. *Thorax*, *61*(10), 833–4.

Page 20 The same areas of our cortex light up like beacons in functional magnetic resonance imaging (fMRI) studies exploring social rejection and emotional hurt as do with physical pain.

Wager, T. D., Atlas, L. Y., Lindquist, M. A., Roy, M., Woo, C. W., & Kross, E. (2013). An fMRI-based neurologic signature of physical pain. *New England Journal of Medicine*, *368*(15), 1388–97.

Page 20 Researchers have noticed that sensations of physical pain can actually be incited by strong negative emotion.

Yarns, B. C., Cassidy, J. T., & Jimenez, A. M. (2022). At the intersection of anger, chronic pain, and the brain: A mini-review. *Neuroscience & Biobehavioral Reviews*, *135*, 104558.

Page 21 Additionally, increased inflammation leads to greater levels of pain

Omoigui, S. (2007). The biochemical origin of pain: the origin of all pain is inflammation and the inflammatory response. Part 2 of 3 - inflammatory profile of pain syndromes. *Medical Hypotheses*. 69(6):1169-78. doi: 10.1016/j.mehy.2007.06.033. Epub 28 Aug. 2007 PMID: 17728071; PMCID: PMC2771434.

Page 21 This separate system can actually operate independently of your brain, with more neurons than the whole of the spinal cord (in the region of 400-600 million).

Fleming, M. A. 2nd, Ehsan., L, Moore, S. R., Levin, D. E., (8 Sep. 2020). The Enteric Nervous System and Its Emerging Role as a Therapeutic Target. Gastroenterol Res Pract. 2020:8024171. doi: 10.1155/2020/8024171. PMID: 32963521; PMCID: PMC7495222.

Page 22 The vagal pathway shares information between our brain and gut via neurotransmitters and hormones (all, in turn, playing a critical role in sleep, stress, pain and mood regulation).
Han, Y., Wang, B., Gao, H., He, C., Hua, R., Liang, C., ... & Xu, J. (2022). Vagus nerve and underlying impact on the gut microbiota-brain axis in behavior and neurodegenerative diseases. *Journal of Inflammation Research, 15*, 6213–30.

Page 22 If this relationship is disrupted by suppressed anger which induces gut symptoms like IBS, these issues then feed back to our brains, and we're stuck in a loop.
Carabotti, M., Scirocco, A., Maselli, M. A., & Severi, C. (2015). The gut–brain axis: Interactions between enteric microbiota, central and enteric nervous systems. *Annals of Gastroenterology: Quarterly Publication of the Hellenic Society of Gastroenterology, 28*(2), 203–9.

Page 22 Just as with reactivity in the gut, our skin can flare with the emotional overload and inverted release of inflammatory elements like anger.
Mento, C., Rizzo, A., Muscatello, M. R. A., Zoccali, R. A., & Bruno, A. (2020). Negative emotions in skin disorders: A systematic review. *International Journal of Psychological Research, 13*(1), 71–86.

Page 23 Certain studies discuss the prevalence of severe hives and psoriasis to the communication of anger.
Altınöz, A. E., Taşkıntuna, N., Altınöz, S. T., Ceran, S. (31 Sep. 2014). A cohort study of the relationship between anger and chronic spontaneous urticaria. *Adv. Ther.* (9):1000-7. doi: 10.1007/s12325-014-0152-6. Epub 2014 Sep 11. PMID: 25209876.

Hughes, O., Hunter, R. (17 Mar. 2022) Understanding the experiences of anger in the onset and progression of psoriasis: A thematic analysis. *Skin Health and Disease* 2(4):e111. doi: 10.1002/ski2.111. PMID: 36479265; PMCID: PMC9720208.

Chapter Four: Girl Baby

Page 32 For starters, there's all the pink. Infants show clear colour preference by at least the age of 12 weeks.
Zemach, I. K., & Teller, D. Y. (2007). Infant color vision: Infants' spontaneous color preferences are well behaved. *Vision Research, 47*(10), 1362–7.

Rippon, G. (2019). *The Gendered Brain*. Vintage.

ENDNOTES

Eliot, L. (2012). *Pink Brain, Blue Brain.* Oneworld Publications.

Page 36 We know that repressed anger may be a perpetuating factor in the pain experience.
Lumley, M. A., Cohen, J. L., Borszcz, G. S., Cano, A., Radcliffe, A. M., Porter, L. S., ... & Keefe, F. J. (2011). Pain and emotion: A biopsychosocial review of recent research. *Journal of Clinical Psychology, 67*(9), 942–68.

Page 38 Recent scientific findings show that people with migraines or tension headaches also present with higher levels of suppressed anger and emotional distress.
Hatch, J. P., Schoenfeld, L. S., Boutros, N. N., Seleshi, E., Moore, P. J., & Cyr-Provost, M. (1991). Anger and hostility in tension-type headache. *Headache: The Journal of Head and Face Pain, 31*(5), 302–4.

Page 38 Frozen carotid wraps around the neck have been noted in trial to significantly diminish migraine pain and were shown by recent meta-analysis to be an instantly effective migraine treatment.
Sprouse-Blum, A. S., Gabriel, A. K., Brown, J. P., & Yee, M. H. (2013). Randomized controlled trial: Targeted neck cooling in the treatment of the migraine patient. *Hawaii Journal of Medicine & Public Health, 72*(7), 237–41.

Page 38 As well as addressing inflammation itself through slowing of blood flow, cold therapy boosts production of both anti-inflammatory products and pro-inflammatory cytokines.
Hsu, Y. Y., Chen, C. J., Wu, S. H., & Chen, K. H. (2023). Cold intervention for relieving migraine symptoms: A systematic review and meta-analysis. *Journal of Clinical Nursing, 32*(11–12), 2455–65.

Page 40 We know that levels of internalised anger are significantly higher in anorexic patients, as compared to control populations.
Horesh, N., Zalsman, G., & Apter, A. (2000). Internalized anger, self-control, and mastery experience in inpatient anorexic adolescents. *Journal of Psychosomatic Research, 49*(4), 247–53.

Page 42 It seems too much of a luxury to open our eyes to the elevated anger scores found in individuals presenting with symptoms of OCD.
Cludius, B., Schmidt, A. F., Moritz, S., Banse, R., & Jelinek, L. (2017). Implicit aggressiveness in patients with obsessive-compulsive disorder as assessed by an Implicit Association Test. *Journal of Behavior Therapy and Experimental Psychiatry, 55*, 106–12.

Radomsky, A. S., Ashbaugh, A. R., & Gelfand, L. A. (2007). Relationships between anger, symptoms, and cognitive factors in OCD checkers. *Behaviour Research and Therapy*, *45*(11), 2712–25.

Chapter Five: Little Girl

Page 53 Not to sound completely joyless (OK, a bit joyless), a recent study involving gender messaging in children's stories proved thought-provoking on the topic of continued teaching of passivity in Little Girls.
Pownall, M., & Heflick, N. (2023). Mr. Active and Little Miss Passive? The transmission and existence of gender stereotypes in children's books. *Sex Roles*, *89*(11), 758–73.

Lewis, M., Cooper Borkenhagen, M., Converse, E., Lupyan, G., & Seidenberg, M. S. (2022). What might books be teaching young children about gender? *Psychological Science*, *33*(1), 33–47.

Page 54 'Stream of consciousness' writing was a concept coined in 1892 by the psychologist William James as a way of accessing the dynamic and covert products of the mind.
James, W. (1892). 'The stream of consciousness.' In: *Psychology*, Chapter XI. Cleveland & New York, World.

Page 55 The fluid home life she was raised in was, in fact, an institution to 'benevolent sexism'.
Barreto, M., & Doyle, D. M. (2023). Benevolent and hostile sexism in a shifting global context. *Nature Reviews Psychology*, *2*(2), 98–111.

Page 59 In Little Girlhood, it's found that families praise male siblings in a different way, which contributes to confidence behaviours later.
Gunderson, E. A., Gripshover, S. J., Romero, C., Dweck, C. S., Goldin-Meadow, S., & Levine, S. C. (2013). Parent praise to 1-to 3-year-olds predicts children's motivational frameworks 5 years later. *Child Development*, *84*(5), 1526–41.

Page 60 As our *passive* Little Girl grows, it makes sense that she might linger too long in more junior roles (in an infantilised, apologetic position) and isn't as far ahead as she could be when she takes maternity leave (during which, male counterparts are receiving promotions).
International Labour Organization (Feb. 2022). The gender gap in employment: What's holding women back? InfoStories. Retrieved from https://www.ilo.org/infostories/en-GB/Stories/Employment/barriers-women#intro.

ENDNOTES

Page 60 A great article by Alena Papayanis in *Huffpost* says it all.
Papayanis, A. (7 Jan. 2022). Women are taught to be nice. Here's what happened when I stopped. HuffPost. Retrieved from https://www.huffpost.com/entry/women-socialized-to-be-nice_n_61d7612be4b04b42ab7d7196.

Page 61 It doesn't matter about the messaging at school, kids learn through observation, from which we deduce patterns about how the world works.
Bouchrika, I. (8 Feb. 2024). Social learning theory & its modern application in education in 2024. Research.com. Retrieved from https://research.com/education/social-learning-theory.

Shukla, A. (4 Dec. 2021). Why did humans evolve pattern recognition abilities? Cognition Today. Retrieved from https://cognitiontoday.com/why-did-humans-evolve-pattern-recognition-abilities/.

Page 62 Nowadays, 41 per cent of UK women work full-time (as opposed to 25 per cent in 2010).
Gov.uk (27 Jul. 2023). Childcare and early years survey of parents. Retrieved from https://explore-education-statistics.service.gov.uk/find-statistics/childcare-and-early-years-survey-of-parents.

Page 62 In the US, it's 37.3 per cent.
Guzman, G., & Kollar, M. (12 Sep. 2023). Income in the United States: 2022. United States Census Bureau. Retrieved from https://www.census.gov/library/publications/2023/demo/p60-279.html#:~:text=In%202022%2C%2065.6%20percent%20of,percent%20between%202021%20and%202022.

Page 62 According to a 2022 article in the *Guardian*, women in heterosexual couples are still completing 65 per cent of the household chores.
Saner, E. (15 Aug. 2022). 'The woman's to-do list is relentless': How to achieve an equal split of household chores. *Guardian*. Retrieved from https://www.theguardian.com/money/2022/aug/15/how-to-achieve-an-equal-split-of-household-chores-kate-mangino.

Page 62 A CBS report suggests that even so-called 'breadwinner' wives spend around three and a half hours more a week than husbands on housework and care provision.
Picchi, A. (13 Apr. 2023). Even 'breadwinner' wives do more housework than husbands.

CBS News. Retrieved from https://www.cbsnews.com/news/women-breadwinners-tripled-since-1970s-still-doing-more-unpaid-work/.

Page 62 'Boys will be boys' is the apparently unshakeable view which sets us up to look at each other differently.
Skipper, Y., & Fox, C. (2022). Boys will be boys: Young people's perceptions and experiences of gender within education. *Pastoral Care in Education*, *40*(4), 391–409.

Page 71 In our first five years of life, billions of neuronal connections are forming.
Rushton, S. (2011). Neuroscience, early childhood education and play: We are doing it right! *Early Childhood Education Journal*, *39*, 89–94.

Page 72 And some babies are just 'higher need' babies with parents who don't have the capacity to accommodate this.
Sears, B. (n.d.). 12 signs your baby is high need. Askdrsears.com. Retrieved from https://www.askdrsears.com/topics/health-concerns/fussy-baby/high-need-baby/12-features-high-need-baby/.

Page 72 I really need to reiterate at this point how plastic (capable of structural reorganisation) our brains are.
Diniz, C. R. A. F., & Crestani, A. P. (2023). The times they are a-changin': A proposal on how brain flexibility goes beyond the obvious to include the concepts of 'upward' and 'downward' to neuroplasticity. *Molecular Psychiatry*, *28*(3), 977–92.

Page 73 Poor Little Girl!
Ferguson, T. J., Stegge, H., Miller, E. R., & Olsen, M. E. (1999). Guilt, shame, and symptoms in children. *Developmental Psychology*, *35*(2), 347–57.

Chapter Six: Tween Girl

Page 77 This is because we've never been granted permission by society, nor a vocabulary, to easily express our angry feelings.
Crofton Winsor, S. (2009). Sugar and spice: The hidden world of pre-adolescent female aggression. Smith College. Retrieved from https://scholarworks.smith.edu/cgi/viewcontent.cgi?article=1524&context=theses.

Page 78 These more sophisticated feelings, which look so far from anger, appear to protect us from the socially destructive expression of pure rage, at a life stage where socially conforming begins to reign supreme.
Moretti, M. M., Catchpole, R. E., & Odgers, C. (2005). The dark side of

girlhood: Recent trends, risk factors and trajectories to aggression and violence. *The Canadian Child and Adolescent Psychiatry Review, 14*(1), 21–5.

Page 78 This is when boys and girls are first divided socially.
Kågesten, A., Gibbs, S., Blum, R. W., Moreau, C., Chandra-Mouli, V., Herbert, A., & Amin, A. (2016). Understanding factors that shape gender attitudes in early adolescence globally: A mixed-methods systematic review. *PloS One, 11*(6), e0157805.

Page 81 If she didn't, she was terrified for her safety (possibly correctly, based on the reported behaviours of her male co-workers on feeling humiliated or rejected).
Acas (15 Mar. 2021). Sexual harassment: What sexual harassment is. Retrieved from https://www.acas.org.uk/sexual-harassment.

Page 85 Zara decided not to mention the relationship to HR, but instead to have a meeting with the perpetrator in a glass room in the middle of the office.
Marks, G. (20 Feb. 2020). Employers can't forbid romance in the workplace – but they can protect workers. *Guardian*. Retrieved from https://www.theguardian.com/business/2020/feb/20/workplace-romances-metoo-rules-protection.

Page 85 Tweenhood is the point at which social media begins to flex its adaptable fingers into the minds of ripely susceptible victims.
Ofcom (29 Mar. 2023). Children and parents: Media use and attitudes 2023. Retrieved from https://www.ofcom.org.uk/__data/assets/pdf_file/0027/255852/childrens-media-use-and-attitudes-report-2023.pdf.

Page 86 The addiction creates further disempowerment and loss of agency, which is disastrous for us women, who might better channel our energy into trying to claw up some substantial power IRL.
Abrams, Z. (3 Aug. 2023). Why young brains are especially vulnerable to social media. American Psychological Association. Retrieved from https://www.apa.org/news/apa/2022/social-media-children-teens.

Page 87 The rift between men and women is written back then in the Tween years, when society muscles in with its crass messaging and boring ideas about boys and girls.
Velding, V. (1 Jan. 2015). Growing up tween: Femininity, masculinity, and coming of age. Wayne State University. Retrieved from https://digitalcommons.wayne.edu/cgi/viewcontent.cgi?article=2352&context=oa_dissertations.

Page 87 The chat, intimacy and maturity encouraged and expected amongst Tween Girls is in opposition to the simplistic rough and tumble of boys' friendships.
Määttä, K., & Uusiautti, S. (2020). Nine contradictory observations about girls' and boys' upbringing and education - the strength-based approach as the way to eliminate the gender gap. *Frontiers in Education*, *5*, 134.

Page 88 This may be as inversions, acts of harm against the self – from repression to actual physical trauma.
Young, R., Van Beinum, M., Sweeting, H., & West, P. (2007). Young people who self-harm. *The British Journal of Psychiatry*, *191*(1), 44–9.

Chapter Seven: Teen Girl

Page 103 Naming assaultive behaviour as such can be alarming to women, particularly if they're younger and haven't yet begun to stand in scrutiny of what they've been socialised to accept.
Bentivegna, F., & Patalay, P. (2022). The impact of sexual violence in mid-adolescence on mental health: A UK population-based longitudinal study. *The Lancet Psychiatry*, *9*(11), 874–83.

Page 103 They're forced to relive the experience again and again, and are themselves held to account and scrutinised.
Murphy-Oikonen, J., McQueen, K., Miller, A., Chambers, L., & Hiebert, A. (2022). Unfounded sexual assault: Women's experiences of not being believed by the police. *Journal of Interpersonal Violence*, *37*(11–12), NP8916–40.

Page 104 Romcoms are structured around the idea of a woman feeling infuriated with, or even disgusted by, a man, only to somehow 'learn' that what she really feels is a deep attraction to him.
Halffield, C. (Apr. 2017). 'She brought it on herself': A discourse analysis of sexual assault in teen comedy film. DePauw University. Retrieved from https://core.ac.uk/download/pdf/214031367.pdf.

Page 104 Through this lens, we can see how diminishing and denigrating this narrative is to her emotions.
Robbins, A. (7 Mar. 2023). Stop normalizing sexual assault in teen movies. Odyssey. Retrieved from https://www.theodysseyonline.com/stop-normalizing-sexual-assault-movies.

ENDNOTES

Page 107 Of course, boys have their issues at this age, but without the baked-in monthly dread that their bodies could feasibly let them down in a way that could be catastrophic to their future selves, socially and academically.
Klass, P. (13 Jan. 2020). When heavy periods disrupt a teenager's life. *New York Times*. Retrieved from https://www.nytimes.com/2020/01/13/well/family/teenagers-heavy-periods-menstrual-cycle-menstruation.html.

Page 110 It was normal.
Department of Psychiatry (1 Jul. 2019). Self-harm in children and adolescents: A major health and social problem of our time. University of Oxford. Retrieved from https://www.psych.ox.ac.uk/news/self-harm-in-children-and-adolescents-a-major-health-and-social-problem-of-our-time.

Page 112 Based on the psychoanalytic idea of wish fulfilment, we might deduce a certain fantasy around her parents' death.
Pataki, T. (2014). *Wish-fulfilment in Philosophy and Psychoanalysis: The tyranny of desire*. Routledge.

Page 114 I hear this a lot – Teen Girl looks so convincingly together and mature, even kind parents can make the mistake of leaving them to it.
Friedersdorf, C. (21 Feb. 2023). Adults are letting teen girls down. *The Atlantic*. Retrieved from https://www.theatlantic.com/newsletters/archive/2023/02/adults-are-letting-teen-girls-down/673144/.

Page 116 This must have only been temporary – which is why it had to run on repeat.
Streep, P. (2 Feb. 2015). 8 toxic patterns in mother–daughter relationships. *Psychology Today*. Retrieved from https://www.psychologytoday.com/gb/blog/tech-support/201502/8-toxic-patterns-in-mother-daughter-relationships.

Page 116 Our minimal prefrontal cortex maturation governs our Teen difficulty with placing ourselves in a wider context.
National Institute of Mental Health (2023). The teen brain: 7 things to know. Retrieved from https://www.nimh.nih.gov/health/publications/the-teen-brain-7-things-to-know#:~:text=The%20brain%20finishes%20developing%20and,prioritizing%2C%20and%20making%20good%20decisions.

Edwards, S. (9 Aug. 2010). Deciphering the teenage brain. Harvard Medical School. Retrieved from https://hms.harvard.edu/news/deciphering-teenage-brain.

Chapter Eight: Young Woman

Page 129 Many psychoanalysts, as well as neuroscientists, would argue that, behaviourally and at a brain developmental level, we're adolescents until we're around 30.
Somerville, L. (2016) Searching for Signatures of Brain Maturity: What Are We Searching For? Neuron (92) 6 pp. 1164-1167

Page 130 Entering into the workplace when our sexual currency is at an all-time high, but our ability to confer respect is at its lowest, is a complex terrain.
Carnegie, M. (20 Jul. 2023). Breaking the office bias: Smashing the workplace stereotypes holding women back. *The Independent.* Retrieved from https://www.independent.co.uk/life-style/galaxy-the-ripple-effect/breaking-bias-workplace-stereotypes-b2366688.html.

Page 130 You wouldn't believe – or maybe you would – the number of Promising Young Women I hear who are careful not to 'reject' affections, so as to protect their place on teams or in supervisors' favours.
TUC (12 May 2023). New TUC poll: 2 in 3 young women have experienced sexual harassment, bullying or verbal abuse at work. Retrieved from https://www.tuc.org.uk/news/new-tuc-poll-2-3-young-women-have-experienced-sexual-harassment-bullying-or-verbal-abuse-work.

Page 130 I'm stunned by the repeated narratives of women patients finding themselves in 'Boys' Club' industries, from advertising to law to tech to film to recruitment to healthcare; lad-ishness, misogyny and mild to appalling levels of harassment are rife.
Powell, K., & Heath, L. (4 Sep. 2023). Beating the business 'boys club': Why there is still so much to be done. Maddyness. Retrieved from https://www.maddyness.com/uk/2023/09/04/beating-the-business-boys-club-why-there-is-still-so-much-to-be-done/.

Page 133 According to the WHO, 1 in 3 pregnant women globally are victims of domestic violence.
Agarwal, S., Prasad, R., Mantri, S., Chandrakar, R., Gupta, S., Babhulkar, V., ... & Wanjari, M. B. (2023). A comprehensive review of intimate partner violence during pregnancy and its adverse effects on maternal and fetal health. *The Cureus Journal of Medical Science, 15*(5), e39262.

ENDNOTES

Page 134 I angled the lens to show her the subtleties of the sado-masochistic system, whereby her training as an Oppressed Person in life – keeping herself in check to others' needs, prioritising their demands, fulfilling the version of her they required – came in very useful.

Fedoroff, J. P. (2008). Sadism, sadomasochism, sex, and violence. *The Canadian Journal of Psychiatry, 53*(10), 637–46.

Page 135 I agreed that, as with any kind of addiction – however the dopamine finds its release – a taste of those neurotransmitters signals to our receptors to search for more.

Johnson, J. L. (3 Jan. 2023). The complex science behind itch in atopic dermatitis. National Eczema Association. Retrieved from https://nationaleczema.org/blog/science-of-itch/#:~:text=Experiencing%20itch%20causes%20the%20desire,of%20pleasure%20associated%20with%20scratching.

Page 137 As it was for our younger selves, there are still few other platforms for women to express their forceful emotions, desires or aggression.

Abrams, A. (23 Feb. 2020). The power and shame of women's anger. *Psychology Today*. Retrieved from https://www.psychologytoday.com/gb/blog/nurturing-self-compassion/202002/the-power-and-shame-women-s-anger.

Page 140 True equality therefore remains a bit of an illusion.

Carrazana, C. (27 Apr. 2023). The 'open secret' in most workplaces: Discrimination against moms is still rampant. The 19th. Retrieved from https://19thnews.org/2023/04/workplace-discrimination-mothers-open-secret/.

Page 143 Possibly because we've been inducted into the importance of keeping a nice home, and the same doesn't seem to have been expected of boys.

Save the Children (n.d.). Gender roles can create lifelong cycle of inequality. Retrieved from https://www.savethechildren.org/us/charity-stories/how-gender-norms-impact-boys-and-girls.

Page 143 For this is when a lifelong, gendered interface with medical institutions really gets going, whether it's for birth control, smear tests, terminations, reproductive issues, endometriosis or yeast infections.

Health and Social Care Services Research (23 Nov. 2022). Women's health: Why do women feel unheard? National Institute for Health and Care Research. Retrieved from https://evidence.nihr.ac.uk/collection/womens-health-why-women-feel-unheard/.

Page 143 Here in the UK, a recent chancellor reallocated a tax of a quarter of a million, levied from tampon sales, into a pro-life organisation.
Britton, A. (29 Oct. 2017). Anti-abortion charity to receive money from tampon tax. *The Independent*. Retrieved from https://www.independent.co.uk/news/uk/politics/tampon-tax-anti-abortion-group-towels-a8025851.html.

Page 144 Consider the enduring issues around menopause medication – shortages, reluctance to prescribe, insistence on blood testing and the paucity of training amongst GPs who are tasked with providing it.
The Menopause Charity (n.d.). How to ask your GP for help. Retrieved from https://www.themenopausecharity.org/wp-content/uploads/2021/05/How-to-ask-your-GP-for-help-rev.pdf.

Page 145 Beginning with the fact that contemporary medical school textbooks don't even include a realistic representation of normal female genitalia, perhaps?
Hayes, J. A. & Temple-Smith, M. J. (2022). New Context, New Content: Rethinking Genital Anatomy in Textbooks in Anatomical Sciences Education, Volume 15, Issue 5 pp. 943-956

Page 146 It's also to do with feeling our bodies themselves are too much.
Jain, P., & Bruzek, L. (10 Jun. 2022). In a world built for men, we don't know much about women's bodies. *Fortune*. Retrieved from https://fortune.com/2022/06/10/world-built-for-men-women-bodies-gender-gap-health-research-medicine-care-jain-bruzek/.

Page 147 Historically, the discourse around infertility and miscarriage has firmly placed accountability at the woman's door, in spite of increasing knowledge that 50 per cent of cases related to infertility are male.
Newcastle University (10 Jan. 2022). Breakthrough into the cause of male infertility. Retrieved from https://www.ncl.ac.uk/press/articles/archive/2022/01/maleinfertilitystudy/#:~:text=It%20is%20estimated%20that%20up,cases%2C%20the%20cause%20is%20unexplained.

Page 147 And that possible damaged DNA and the more general health of sperm is becoming a more widely researched area.
Wighton, K. (4 Jan. 2019). Recurrent miscarriage linked to faulty sperm. Imperial College London. Retrieved from https://www.imperial.ac.uk/news/189690/recurrent-miscarriage-linked-faulty-sperm/.

ENDNOTES

Alahmar, A. T., Singh, R., & Palani, A. (2022). Sperm DNA fragmentation in reproductive medicine: A review. *Journal of Human Reproductive Sciences*, *15*(3), 206–18.

Page 147 Nonetheless, historical implication and imagination identifies the woman's body as the suspect, which, still today, often means a woman doesn't allow herself a real experience of grief if she miscarries.

Bello, C. (10 Jun. 2023). Fertility is not just a 'women's problem' but a fifth of men think it is, a new study finds. Euronews. Retrieved from https://www.euronews.com/health/2023/06/10/fertility-is-not-just-a-womens-problem-yet-a-fifth-of-men-think-it-is-study-finds.

Bueno, J. (22 Jun. 2019). Why do women blame themselves after miscarriage? *Psychology Today*. Retrieved from https://www.psychologytoday.com/gb/blog/the-brink-being/201906/why-do-women-blame-themselves-after-miscarriage.

Page 153 A note around money for the Young Woman: get this sorted. I find myself struck – again – by an atmosphere of the fifties, as women describe to me that the husband manages all the money and accounts and that she 'doesn't really know what's going on'.

Hanna, S. D., Kim, K. T., Lindamood, S., & Lee, S. T. (2021). Husbands, wives, and financial knowledge in wealthy households. *Financial Planning Review*, *4*(1), e1110.

Page 153 According to the Duluth 'Power and Control Wheel', which denotes categories of financial abuse, giving someone an allowance/not allowing access to family income registers high as a predictor of power imbalance.

Domestic Abuse Intervention Programs (n.d.). Wheel information center. Retrieved from https://www.theduluthmodel.org/wheels/.

Page 154 But, as yet, the experience of women delivering stillborn babies doesn't seem to have come under as-active scrutiny.

Hopkins Leisher, S. (4 Nov. 2020). Stillbirth leaves millions suffering in silence – we must do more to prevent it and end the stigma. *Telegraph*. Retrieved from https://www.telegraph.co.uk/global-health/women-and-girls/stillbirth-leaves-millions-suffering-silence-must-do-prevent/?WT.mc_id=tmgoff_psc_ppc_performancemax_dynamiclandingpages&gclid=CjwKCAjwvfmoBhAwEiwAG2tqzHjO8u4_VAlOyxybGxcaroty6dHW-lXwcfp2uCxqYltzFS_wVx1ykRoCX0UQAvD_BwE.

WOMEN ARE <u>ANGRY</u>

Page 154 Though there are offers of counselling, if 'she would like', a counsellor needs to come in and take the hand of this woman – she doesn't have the means to get herself into *their* room.
Kelley, M. C., & Trinidad, S. B. (2012). Silent loss and the clinical encounter: Parents' and physicians' experiences of stillbirth – a qualitative analysis. *BMC Pregnancy and Childbirth*, 12, 137.

Page 155 The Royal College of Obstetricians and Gynaecologists discusses the importance of giving birth naturally to a dead baby for the woman's physical health, and for the health of future births.
Royal College of Obstetricians & Gynaecologists (Feb. 2019). When your baby dies before birth. Retrieved from https://www.rcog.org.uk/for-the-public/browse-our-patient-information/when-your-baby-dies-before-birth/.

Page 155 But, time and again, it occurs to me that the psychological impact is seemingly underconsidered, which doesn't get addressed, because how would a woman be able to leave 'feedback'?
Cena, L., & Stefana, A. (2020). Psychoanalytic perspectives on the psychological effects of stillbirth on parents: A protocol for systematic review and qualitative synthesis. *Frontiers in Psychology*, 11, 1216.

Page 155 Young Woman begins to understand, even if only in her unconscious, that the field of medicine, populated exclusively by men until the twenty-first century, has left an unquestioned legacy in its wake concerning the female experience; their needs, their mental health.
Leonard, J. (17 Jun. 2021). Gender bias in medical diagnosis. Medical News Today. Retrieved from https://www.medicalnewstoday.com/articles/gender-bias-in-medical-diagnosis#what-are-the-causes.

Page 156 Over here, women's health is under-researched and under resourced.
Bird, C. (11 Feb. 2022). Underfunding of research in women's health issues is the biggest missed opportunity in health care. RAND. Retrieved from https://www.rand.org/pubs/commentary/2022/02/underfunding-of-research-in-womens-health-issues-is.html.

Winchester, N. (1 Jul. 2021). Women's health outcomes: Is there a gender gap? House of Lords Library. Retrieved from https://lordslibrary.parliament.uk/womens-health-outcomes-is-there-a-gender-gap/.

ENDNOTES

Page 157 Midwife-led or homecare certainly seem to provide more natural-seeming solutions.
NHS (8 Apr. 2021). Where to give birth: The options. Retrieved from https://www.nhs.uk/pregnancy/labour-and-birth/preparing-for-the-birth/where-to-give-birth-the-options/.

Page 157 But, in reality, understaffing can make these options dangerous and create trauma around unplanned intervention.
Baby Loss and Maternity All Party Parliamentary Groups (Oct. 2022). Safe staffing: The impact of staffing shortages in maternity and neonatal care. Sands. Retrieved from https://www.sands.org.uk/sites/default/files/Staffing%20shortages%20-%20APPG%20report,%20Oct%2022%20(final).pdf.

Page 157 I worry that, again, tokenistic provision of birthing centres, if they can't be safely staffed, leaves women feeling less in control and more exposed to danger.
Linton, D. (14 Feb. 2022). 'The maternity ward felt dangerous – we were so short-staffed I had to work after my miscarriage.' *Telegraph*. Retrieved from https://www.telegraph.co.uk/health-fitness/body/maternity-ward-felt-dangerous-short-staffed-had-work-miscarriage/.

Page 157 The dearth of financial support and academic research into issues affecting women, from childbirth to menopause to fibromyalgia, betrays the classically dismal view of services which would benefit women's health and actually help them contribute revenue.
Graham, S. (16 Mar. 2021). Women are still branded 'hysterical' because of chronic illnesses which are under-researched and under-funded. *inews*. Retrieved from https://inews.co.uk/opinion/chronic-illness-women-me-fibromyalgia-research-treatment-905879.

Onarheim, K. H., Iversen, J. H., & Bloom, D. E. (2016). Economic benefits of investing in women's health: A systematic review. *PloS One*, *11*(3), e0150120.

Page 157 Horrifying findings in the media bear out the tendency towards ignoring what women are telling professionals about their own bodies.
Wellbeing of Women (15 Nov. 2022). Over half of UK women feel their pain is ignored or dismissed, new report shows. Retrieved from https://www.wellbeingofwomen.org.uk/news/over-half-of-uk-women-feel-their-pain-is-ignored-or-dismissed-new-report-shows/.

Northwell Health (n.d.). Gaslighting in women's health: No, it's not just in your head. Retrieved from https://www.northwell.edu/katz-institute-for-womens-health/articles/gaslighting-in-womens-health.

Page 159 From where I sit, this looks bleak.
Home Affairs Committee (12 Apr. 2022). Investigation and prosecution of rape – Report summary. UK Parliament. Retrieved from https://publications.parliament.uk/pa/cm5802/cmselect/cmhaff/193/summary.html

Page 159 A process presided over and legislated by men can never hope to provide the neutrality and safety required by a woman publicly exposing herself through trial.
Mahdawi, A. (2 Oct. 2021). The US criminal justice system is failing sexual assault survivors. It needs a feminist overhaul. *Guardian*. Retrieved from https://www.theguardian.com/commentisfree/2021/oct/02/us-criminal-justice-system-failing-sexual-assault-survivors-feminist-overhaul.

Page 161 How can women's bodies and experiences still be treated so disdainfully?
Bhatia, S. (13 Dec. 2021). 'What were you wearing?' – How the criminal justice system is failing to deliver access to justice for women who are victims of sexual assault and rape. The official blog of the UCL Centre for Access to Justice and Student Pro Bono Committee. Retrieved from https://reflect.ucl.ac.uk/access-to-justice/2021/12/13/what-were-you-wearing-how-the-criminal-justice-system-is-failing-to-deliver-access-to-justice-for-women-who-are-victims-of-sexual-assault-and-rape/.

Page 163 Support other women as a first reflex. That instinct is data-backed.
Rape Crisis England & Wales (5 Oct. 2022). Our comment on granting suspects anonymity. Retrieved from https://rapecrisis.org.uk/news/our-comment-on-granting-suspects-anonymity/.

Chapter Nine: Adult Woman

Page 165 Many certainly seem very busy.
Dunn, J. (17 May 2023). What to do about uninvolved grandparents. Parents.com. Retrieved from https://www.parents.com/parenting/dynamics/grandparents/uninvolved-grandparents/.

ENDNOTES

Page 165 Or are located far away because trying to Have It All meant that Adult Woman might live in a city she didn't grow up in.

Anon. (2 Jan. 2023). My parents are too busy to be grandparents. *Telegraph*. Retrieved from https://www.telegraph.co.uk/family/parenting/parents-busy-grandparents/?WT.mc_id=tmgoff_psc_ppc_performancemax_dynamiclandingpages&gclid=CjwKCAjw-KipBhBtEiwAWjgwrKpLDgHcvMSDbzxGrJ5tO-PbBXb62rWCZzwrOfF8n5kj7a9Diso9ghoClxMQAvD_BwE.

Page 165 She may have had to move for her partner's work or perhaps those parents might now be a bit too old to help.

Guardian (19 Aug. 2017). A letter to … my in-laws, who are apathetic grandparents. Retrieved from https://www.theguardian.com/lifeandstyle/2017/aug/19/a-letter-to-my-in-laws-who-are-apathetic-grandparents.

Page 165 From navigating a health system stacked against her to returning to career 'proper' after maternity leaves, sleep-deprived and glued together with milky vomit and nappy cream, yes, indeed, Adult Woman is where I see female rage at arguably its supercharged, its most visceral – and at its most sublimated and physicalised.

Ou, C. H., Hall, W. A., Rodney, P., & Stremler, R. (2022). Seeing red: A grounded theory study of women's anger after childbirth. *Qualitative Health Research*, *32*(12), 1780–94.

Page 166 Hitting the glass ceilings, crashing headlong into absurd inequality and tasting the futility of a circular system are de rigueur across the Reproductive Years – mirroring the extent to which our hands are tied to do much about it.

Alhosseiny, H. (2023). Glass-ceiling: The never-ending anguish of working women. *Journal of Entrepreneurship Education*, *26*(S3), 1–12.

Page 166 Typically, we bury the rage deep inside and watch it emerge as a host of different symptoms.

Thomas, S. P. (2005). Women's anger, aggression, and violence. *Health Care for Women International*, *26*(6), 504–22.

Page 166 Whilst it's undeniable that women's neurology changes on childbirth, I believe that patriarchal structures exploit those biological events.

Duarte-Guterman, P., Leuner, B., & Galea, L. A. (2019). The long and short term effects of motherhood on the brain. *Frontiers in Neuroendocrinology*, *53*, 100740.

Page 167 And, as we've seen, we've been primed to carry it since before we were born.
Reich-Stiebert, N., Froehlich, L., & Voltmer, J. B. (2023). Gendered mental labor: A systematic literature review on the cognitive dimension of unpaid work within the household and childcare. *Sex Roles, 88*(11), 475–94.

Page 167 A frightening number of women come to me telling me that their professions have had to go as a result of the demands of mothering.
Artz, B., Kaya, I., & Kaya, O. (2022). Gender role perspectives and job burnout. *Review of Economics of the Household, 20*(2), 447–70.

Page 167 In psychology, we're taught to view problems through the lens of the biopsychosocial.
PsychDB (27 Jan. 2024). Biopsychosocial model and case formulation . Retrieved from https://www.psychdb.com/teaching/biopsychosocial-case-formulation.

Page 168 Which, for men, may mean that more ownership for this shared state needs to be accepted.
Regus, P. (3 Aug. 2007). The emerging medicalization of postpartum depression: Tightening the boundaries of motherhood. Georgia State University. Retrieved from https://scholarworks.gsu.edu/cgi/viewcontent. cgi?article=1015&context=sociology_theses.

Page 169 The danger with terming feelings of impotent rage around new motherhood 'postnatal depression' is that it lets off the hook those around you – the people who apparently were so thrilled about you providing them with a son/daughter/niece/nephew/grandson/grandchild.
Cho, H., Lee, K., Choi, E., Cho, H. N., Park, B., Suh, M., ... & Choi, K. S. (2022). Association between social support and postpartum depression. *Scientific Reports, 12*(1), 3128.

Page 169 The brain registering the near-death experience of childbirth as trauma is entirely plausible.
NCT (Jul. 2022). Traumatic birth and post-traumatic stress disorder. Retrieved from https://www.nct.org.uk/labour-birth/you-after-birth/traumatic-birth-and-post-traumatic-stress-disorder.

ENDNOTES

Page 169 Up to 45 per cent of women experience it that way; waking up sweating in the night, flashbacks, panic attacks.
Beck, C. T., Watson, S., & Gable, R. K. (2018). Traumatic childbirth and its aftermath: Is there anything positive? *The Journal of Perinatal Education, 27*(3), 175–84.

Page 171 I have a sense from where I sit that this tendency is growing.
Thombs, B. D., Levis, B., Lyubenova, A., Neupane, D., Negeri, Z., Wu, Y., ... & Benedetti, A. (2020). Overestimation of postpartum depression prevalence based on a 5-item version of the EPDS: Systematic review and individual participant data meta-analysis. *The Canadian Journal of Psychiatry, 65*(12), 835–44.

Page 171 The apparently 'skewed' numbers during the pandemic, where new mums were reported twice as likely to suffer, were revealing and truthful.
UCL (11 May 2021). New mothers twice as likely to have post-natal depression in lockdown. Retrieved from https://www.ucl.ac.uk/news/2021/may/new-mothers-twice-likely-have-post-natal-depression-lockdown.

Page 171 What my female patient now sees, when she becomes Mother, is that she quickly risks losing her hard-won stake in society.
The Economist (15 Dec. 2018). Why so little is done to help new mums cope. Retrieved from https://www.economist.com/international/2018/12/15/why-so-little-is-done-to-help-new-mums-cope?utm_medium=cpc.adword.pd&utm_source=google&ppccampaignID=18156330227&ppcadID=&utm_campaign=a.22brand_pmax&utm_content=conversion.direct-response.anonymous&gclid=Cj0KCQjwpompBhDZARIsAFD_Fp8LQit21t55AAjfv14Vn6NO8nlAdmYAGuuvJyCUNuNojno7aD5OFz8aAg8hEALw_wcB&gclsrc=aw.ds.

Page 172 For many Adult Women, maternity leave means taking a financial hit.
Almond, D., Cheng, Y., & Machado, C. (2023). Large motherhood penalties in US administrative microdata. *Proceedings of the National Academy of Sciences, 120*(29), e2209740120.

Page 172 These women patients report a huge feeling of discomfort at no longer holding a financial stake, at being placed in a position which means they have to ask for money or are given an allowance by their husbands (allowances, to remind you, are legally classed as abusive).
Keynes, S. (8 Sep. 2023). Motherhood is full of surprises – the economic ones sting the most. *Financial Times*. Retrieved from https://www.ft.com/content/8fcb72d2-d36f-4c60-8a2a-c97d76773bbb.

WOMEN ARE <u>ANGRY</u>

Page 172 This can bring pressures and tensions into a relationship which I feel are really The Voice of Patriarchy, as much as they're anything to do specifically with the couple themselves. If one woman spends a lifetime losing out, two women lose out in ways which are difficult to properly quantify.
Schneebaum, A., & Badgett, M. L. (2019). Poverty in US lesbian and gay couple households. *Feminist Economics*, *25*(1), 1–30.

Zandri, P. (15 Aug. 2023). Are women financially worse off than men after divorce? LinkedIn. Retrieved from https://www.linkedin.com/pulse/women-financially-worse-off-than-men-after-divorce-paige-zandri/.

Page 172 With many women waiting until their thirties before having their first baby (cruising for that *geriatric pregnancy* ...), it could be argued that she *is* lucky – and pitted against the pain of childlessness when a baby is so desperately desired, these complex postpartum feelings can seem at best spoilt and at worst heinous.
Office for National Statistics (27 Jan. 2022). Childbearing for women born in different years, England and Wales: 2020. Retrieved from https://www.ons.gov.uk/peoplepopulationandcommunity/birthsdeathsandmarriages/conceptionandfertilityrates/bulletins/childbearingforwomenbornindifferentyearsenglandandwales/2020.

Page 173 And, by now, we know what happens to internalised rage ...
Billotte Verhoff, C., Hosek, A. M., & Cherry, J. (2023). 'A fire in my belly:' Conceptualizing US women's experiences of 'mom rage'. *Sex Roles*, *88*(11–12), 495–513.

Page 173 And because we're allegedly now so in charge of our bodies and fertility that she can't argue this baby was a surprise, it seems outrageous that she should be experiencing any divergent feelings when said baby arrives, which contributes to the frequently cheated, enraged and ashamed feelings I hear about.
Meeussen, L., & Van Laar, C. (2018). Feeling pressure to be a perfect mother relates to parental burnout and career ambitions. *Frontiers in Psychology*, *9*, 342086.

Page 178 When we team up with others going through something similar, that sense of meaning and connectedness we're longing for can begin to seed.
Cramer, K. M., & Pawsey, H. (2023). Happiness and sense of community belonging in the world value survey. *Current Research in Ecological and Social Psychology*, *4*, 100101.

ENDNOTES

Page 180 If a marriage or partnership ultimately breaks down (which we know the poor division of The Load contributes to), watch how many husbands change their childcare days and stretch the arrangement and gaslight around custody agreements to suit themselves – even schedules which have been drawn up in the courts.

Parker, G., Durante, K. M., Hill, S. E., & Haselton, M. G. (2022). Why women choose divorce: An evolutionary perspective. *Current Opinion in Psychology*, *43*, 300–6.

Page 181 Women are punished both outside and inside the institution of marriage.

American Sociological Association (22 Aug. 2015). Women more likely than men to initiate divorces, but not non-marital breakups. Retrieved from https://www. asanet.org/women-more-likely-men-initiate-divorces-not-non-marital-breakups/.

Page 181 When inside of the institution which is meant to protect her so well, the expectation that women will arrange gifts and remember her partner's family birthdays also seems normalised.

Niedźwieńska, A., & Zielińska, M. (2021). Gender differences in remembering about things to do depend on partnership status. *Sex Roles*, *84*(3), 139–51.

Page 182 This meant his wife had to 'speed up', and was herself now suffering the medical repercussions of this – namely, raised blood pressure and the whisperings of an irregular heartbeat.

Buckley, U., & Shivkumar, K. (2016). Stress-induced cardiac arrhythmias: The heart–brain interaction. *Trends in Cardiovascular Medicine*, *26*(1), 78–80.

Page 182 And frightened men are often aggressive men.

Monbiot, G. (16 Jan. 2019). The fear that lies behind aggressive masculinity. *Guardian*. Retrieved from https://www.theguardian.com/commentisfree/2019/jan/16/men-masculinity-gillette-advertisement.

Page 184 When she arrived in my consulting room, Bianca had recently been diagnosed with fibromyalgia.

Galvez-Sánchez, C. M., Reyes del Paso, G. A., Duschek, S., & Montoro, C. I. (2022). The link between fibromyalgia syndrome and anger: A systematic review revealing research gaps. *Journal of Clinical Medicine*, *11*(3), 844.

Page 187 Society does this to all of us – and then pits us against each other, as we try to crawl through the quagmire of various conditioning.
Kiner, M. (14 Apr. 2020). It's time to break the cycle of female rivalry. *Harvard Business Review*. Retrieved from https://hbr.org/2020/04/its-time-to-break-the-cycle-of-female-rivalry.

Page 188 Male DNA has been identified in the female brain, suggesting that little bits of her son are lodged permanently in the brain of his mother.
Chan, W. F., Gurnot, C., Montine, T. J., Sonnen, J. A., Guthrie, K. A., & Nelson, J. L. (2012). Male microchimerism in the human female brain. *PLoS One*, 7(9), e45592.

Page 188 This has implications for her body as it ages, in terms of certain vulnerabilities to disease.
Relton, C. L. (2014). What is it about boys? *International Journal of Epidemiology*, 43(1), 5–7.

Page 189 Perversely, it's also the mother who misses the promotions and faces streamlining and redundancy drives, and doesn't have much of a leg to stand on, when those around her are able to appear so easily committed and unconstrained.
Jarvis, D. (19 May 2023). Employers must stop penalising women for having children. *New Statesman*. Retrieved from https://www.newstatesman.com/spotlight/economic-growth/cost-of-living-crisis/2023/05/employers-penalising-women-children-pregnancy-redundancy-bill.

Page 191 Since 95 per cent of serotonin is produced in the gut, it makes sense that this is where the hollow is felt.
Appleton, J. (2018). The gut–brain axis: Influence of microbiota on mood and mental health. *Integrative Medicine: A Clinician's Journal*, 17(4), 28–32.

Page 194 Worse still, is the way women end up acclimating to the loss of true equality and partnership in their relationship when babies come along.
Morgan, K. (22 Jun. 2023) Why many women prioritise their partners' jobs. BBC Worklife. Retrieved from https://www.bbc.com/worklife/article/20230620-why-many-women-prioritise-their-partners-jobs.

ENDNOTES

Page 195 This subtle denigration and exploitation becomes evidence of exactly that ordinary, invisible violation of Adult Woman we're talking about.
UN Women (n.d.). FAQs: Types of violence against women and girls. Retrieved from https://www.unwomen.org/en/what-we-do/ending-violence-against-women/faqs/types-of-violence.

Page 196 In 2020, the equivalent of 11 women and girls every minute lost their lives to someone in their family.
United Nations (n.d.). UNODC Research: 2020 saw a woman or girl being killed by someone in their family every 11 minutes. Retrieved from https://www.unodc.org/unodc/frontpage/2021/November/unodc-research_-2020-saw-every-11-minutes-a-woman-or-girl-being-killed-by-someone-in-their-family.html.

Page 196 We also need to remember that half of cases are never reported.
European Institute for Gender Equality (21 Nov. 2017). Gender Equality Index 2017: We cannot be silent about violence. Retrieved from https://eige.europa.eu/news/gender-equality-index-2017-we-cannot-be-silent-about-violence.

Page 197 It takes a different kind of man – an emotionally stronger man, perhaps one who himself has had some therapy – to allow a woman this opportunity to flourish in her multiple roles, and not feel intimidated and crushed by her growth.
Pappas, S. (2019). APA issues first-ever guidelines for practice with men and boys. American Psychological Association. Retrieved from https://www.apa.org/monitor/2019/01/ce-corner.

Page 199 I found myself giggling recently about a Scottish parliamentary apology to women of the 1600s who had lost their lives after having been accused of witchcraft.
Cramer, M. (9 Mar. 2022). Scotland apologizes for history of witchcraft persecution. *New York Times*. Retrieved from https://www.nytimes.com/2022/03/09/world/europe/scotland-nicola-sturgeon-apologizes-witches.html#:~:text=Nicola%20Sturgeon%2C%20the%20first%20minister,the%2016th%20and%2018th%20centuries.

Page 200 The neuroendocrine dysregulation brought on by carting extreme negative emotion around internally has been connected with the development of several chronic illnesses, and even earlier mortality.
Chapman, B. P., Fiscella, K., Kawachi, I., Duberstein, P., & Muennig, P. (2013). Emotion suppression and mortality risk over a 12-year follow-up. *Journal of Psychosomatic Research, 75*(4), 178.

Korte, S. M., Koolhaas, J. M., Wingfield, J. C., & McEwen, B. S. (2005). The Darwinian concept of stress: Benefits of allostasis and costs of allostatic load and the trade-offs in health and disease. *Neuroscience & Biobehavioral Reviews*, *29*(1), 3–38.

Page 202 Why aren't more of you offering shared paternity leave which enables fathers to live off the income?
Topping, A. (26 Apr. 2021). Shared parental leave: Scrap 'deeply flawed' policy, say campaigners. *Guardian*. Retrieved from https://www.theguardian.com/money/2021/apr/26/shared-parental-leave-scrap-deeply-flawed-policy-say-campaigners.

Chapter Ten: Menopausal Woman

Page 205 'Where have all the women gone?' is a repeated refrain across financial districts, the law sector, senior management roles and exec boards.
Wichert, I. (2011). *Where Have All The Senior Women Gone?* Palgrave Macmillan.

Bamford, A. (8 Mar. 2023). 'Where have the women gone?': Exploring industry equality. Design Week. Retrieved from https://www.designweek.co.uk/issues/6-march-10-march-2023/international-womens-day-exploring-industry-equality/.

Page 205 According to the UK Parliament's First Report of Session 2022–23 on Menopause and the Workplace, a BUPA survey found that 900,000 women had quit their jobs due to unmanageable experiences of menopause.
Women and Equalities Committee (28 Jul. 2022). Menopause and the workplace. UK Parliament. Retrieved from https://publications.parliament.uk/pa/cm5803/cmselect/cmwomeq/91/report.html.

Page 205 Nonetheless, employers recognise the brain drain of wisdom and expertise brought about by the mass exodus of, historically, only recently-arrived female employees who've responded to a mix of internal and external cues to shuffle off into the wings.
Treasury Committee (22 Mar. 2010). Women in the City – Tenth report. House of Commons. Retrieved from https://publications.parliament.uk/pa/cm200910/cmselect/cmtreasy/482/48202.htm.

Page 206 This isn't helped by the fabled Queen Bee syndrome, where female bosses are found to treat younger female employees differently.
Ellemers, N., Van den Heuvel, H., De Gilder, D., Maass, A., & Bonvini, A. (2004). The underrepresentation of women in science: Differential commitment or the queen bee syndrome? *British Journal of Social Psychology*, *43*(3), 315–38.

ENDNOTES

Page 206 Researchers tend to feel this is potentially connected to the senior colleague's own knowledge of what it took to get them there and their concern that other women *should* commit, or would be capable of committing in this way.

Elsesser, K. (31 Aug. 2020). Queen bees still exist, but it's not the women we need to fix. *Forbes*. Retrieved from https://www.forbes.com/sites/kimelsesser/2020/08/31/queen-bees-still-exist-but-its-not-the-women-we-need-to-fix/?sh=1358767e6ffd.

Page 208 Many women discuss their problems with the coil, whether copper or hormonal.

Sinha, R., & Singh, S. K. (2020). Migrated intrauterine contraceptive device into urinary bladder and peritoneal cavity: A friend turned foe if forgotten. *International Journal of Clinical Obstetrics and Gynaecology*, 4(2A), 29–31.

Page 208 Power, when shared more equally, actually has the capacity to benefit everyone widely.

UN Women (feb. 2024). Facts and figures: Economic empowerment. Retrieved from https://www.unwomen.org/en/what-we-do/economic-empowerment/facts-and-figures.

Page 208 Because it's such a relatively cheap and effective way of treating a multitude of conditions, and because so many women do get on so well with it, there's a sense of the silver bullet around it.

Lanzola, E. L., & Ketvertis, K. (2022). Intrauterine device. *StatPearls* [internet]. Retrieved from https://www.ncbi.nlm.nih.gov/books/NBK557403/

Page 209 But there's an air of dismissal and, if you're awkward to help, a definite sense you're made to feel it.

balance by Newson Health (13 Oct. 2021). My doctor won't budge! – Shared decision making with your healthcare professional. Retrieved from https://www.balance-menopause.com/menopause-library/my-doctor-wont-budge-shared-decision-making-with-your-healthcare-professional/

Page 212 Together, they discovered that repeated urinary tract infections were the source of her problem.

Hui, C. K. (2014). Recurrent extended-spectrum beta-lactamase-producing Escherichia coli urinary tract infection due to an infected intrauterine device. *Singapore Medical Journal*, 55(2), e28–30.

WOMEN ARE <u>ANGRY</u>

Page 212 They decided the IUD may not be the best thing for her and, together, planned a different package of care.
https://thebms.org.uk/wp-content/uploads/2022/01/HRT-Equivalent-preparations-7th-January-22.pdf

Page 216 This strikes a similar note to the women in roles of leadership and authority I work with clinically, who report feeling squashed by pressures to be so much to so many, and still feel they haven't 'won'.
Ro, C. (19 Jan. 2021). Why do we still distrust women leaders? BBC Worklife. Retrieved from https://www.bbc.com/worklife/article/20210108-why-do-we-still-distrust-women-leaders.

Page 216 From the other side, it can look as if females in positions of seniority seem impelled to treat other women badly; patronising, bullying and frequently unsupportive of mothers, denigrated by their male colleagues and subordinates, and reviled by women employees.
Ade, Y. (31 Jan. 2022). Genuine reasons why some women don't want female bosses. Medium. Retrieved from https://aninjusticemag.com/genuine-reasons-why-some-women-dont-want-female-bosses-df9524058c.

Cosmopolitan (6 Mar. 2014). Why are we so hard on women bosses? Retrieved from https://www.cosmopolitan.com/career/advice/a5872/women-bosses/.

Page 218 As we saw earlier, inflammation is linked to chronic levels of anger.
Pederson, T. Intermittent explosive disorder: Anger disorder linked to inflammation. Accessed December 11, 2017.

Page 218 It also provides a favourable environment for tumour formation and metastasis.
Zhao, H., Wu, L., Yan, G., Chen, Y., Zhou, M., Wu, Y., & Li, Y. (2021). Inflammation and tumor progression: Signaling pathways and targeted intervention. *Signal Transduction and Targeted Therapy*, 6(1), 263.

Page 218 For example, chronic inflammatory bowel diseases, such as ulcerative colitis, carry an increased risk of colon cancer.
National Cancer Institute (29 Apr. 2015). Chronic inflammation. Retrieved from https://www.cancer.gov/about-cancer/causes-prevention/risk/chronic-inflammation.

ENDNOTES

Page 219 Copious studies discuss exceptionally low levels of anger amongst cancer patients, leading to the conclusion amongst researchers that anger is being repressed.
Thomas, S. P., Groer, M., Davis, M., Droppleman, P., Mozingo, J., & Pierce, M. (2000). Anger and cancer: An analysis of the linkages. *Journal of Cancer Nursing, 23*(5), 344–9.

Page 219 Significant evidence also points to suppressed anger as a forerunner to cancer, as well as a component in the advancement of cancer, following its onset.
Ibid.

Page 220 Medical science is nowadays vocal about its findings concerning the feedback relationship between brain and gut, between mind and body.
Schächtle, M. A., & Rosshart, S. P. (2021). The microbiota-gut-brain axis in health and disease and its implications for translational research. *Frontiers in Cellular Neuroscience, 15*, 698172.

Page 221 Results from scientific studies suggest a robust association between sleep deprivation and mood, based on the fact that the amygdala is implicated in both.
Saghir, Z., Syeda, J. N., Muhammad, A. S., Abdalla, T. H. B., & Abdalla, T. H. B. (2018). The amygdala, sleep debt, sleep deprivation, and the emotion of anger: A possible connection? *The Cureus Journal of Medical Science, 10*(7).

Page 221 Women fantasise about bowing out of their intense roles at work because they're just so damn tired. Some actually do.
Viotti, S., Guidetti, G., Sottimano, I., Travierso, L., Martini, M., & Converso, D. (2021). Do menopausal symptoms affect the relationship between job demands, work ability, and exhaustion? Testing a moderated mediation model in a sample of Italian administrative employees. *International Journal of Environmental Research and Public Health, 18*(19), 10029.

Page 222 We're reminded by her experiences of how, even at a basic level, everything from our mood to our immune systems are compromised when we don't sleep well, and the extent to which these fundamentals are essential for well-being.
Olsen, E. J. (28 Nov. 2018). Lack of sleep: Can it make you sick? Mayo Clinic. Retrieved from https://www.mayoclinic.org/diseases-conditions/insomnia/expert-answers/lack-of-sleep/faq-20057757#:~:text=Certain%20cytokines%20need%20to%20increase,don%27t%20get%20enough%20sleep.

Page 222 We need to sleep for our bodies to deal with inflammation, and we also need it for our emotional immunity.
D'Acquisto, F. (2017). Affective immunology: Where emotions and the immune response converge. *Dialogues in Clinical Neuroscience, 19*(1), 9–19.

Page 225 Some still insist on testing hormone levels, which we know is not useful, since levels constantly fluctuate.
British Menopause Society (2022). NICE: Menopause, diagnosis and management – from guideline to practice. Retrieved from https://thebms.org.uk/wp-content/uploads/2022/12/09-BMS-TfC-NICE-Menopause-Diagnosis-and-Management-from-Guideline-to-Practice-Guideline-Summary-NOV2022-A.pdf.

Page 227 Evidence is established that long-distance walking can ease psychological distress, and we know that the bi-lateral movement of walking is emotionally reparative.
Mau, M., Aaby, A., Klausen, S. H., & Roessler, K. K. (2021). Are long-distance walks therapeutic? A systematic scoping review of the conceptualization of long-distance walking and its relation to mental health. *International Journal of Environmental Research and Public Health, 18*(15), 7741.

Diamond, M. (2016). The physical and mental health benefits of walking. Imperial Health + Wellbeing. Retrieved from https://www.imperialhealthatwork.co.uk/blog/2016/1/27/the-physical-and-mental-health-benefits-of-walking#:~:text=The%20natural%2C%20rhythmic%2C%20side%2D,healing%20from%20issues%20such%20as.

Page 227 Research points to a reduction in amygdala activity even after an hour's walking.
Sudimac, S., Sale, V., & Kühn, S. (2022). How nature nurtures: Amygdala activity decreases as the result of a one-hour walk in nature. *Molecular Psychiatry, 27*(11), 4446–52.

Chapter Eleven: Older Woman

Page 231 For starters, Older Woman is more likely to face neglect and abuse.
United Nations (2013). Neglect, abuse and violence against older women. Retrieved from https://www.un.org/esa/socdev/documents/ageing/neglect-abuse-violence-older-women.pdf.

ENDNOTES

Page 231 We're also the ones stuck with enduring either a lonely, cold old age or caring for an ailing husband.
Centre for Ageing Better (26 Nov. 2020). Later life prospects for women much worse than for men, report warns. Retrieved from https://ageing-better.org.uk/news/later-life-prospects-women-much-worse-men-report-warns.

Page 231 Older female workers are twice as likely as men to be carers, according to UK Census 2021.
https://www.ons.gov.uk/peoplepopulationandcommunity/birthsdeathsandmarriages/ageing/articles/livinglongerhowourpopulationischangingandwhyitmatters/2019-03-15

Page 231 A 2022 study clearly demonstrated that caregivers of men were 'more likely to be distressed, remain distressed or become distressed within one year'.
Li, W., Manuel, D. G., Isenberg, S. R., & Tanuseputro, P. (2022). Caring for older men and women: Whose caregivers are more distressed? A population-based retrospective cohort study. *BMC Geriatrics, 22*(1), 890.

Page 232 Interestingly, Older Woman herself is more likely to be denied healthcare, since she's often seen as too fragile to cope with treatment effects.
Chrisler, J. C., Barney, A., & Palatino, B. (2016). Ageism can be hazardous to women's health: Ageism, sexism, and stereotypes of older women in the healthcare system. *Journal of Social Issues, 72*(1), 86–104.

Page 232 She's also at increased risk of exclusion and poverty in old age.
https://eige.europa.eu/publications-resources/toolkits-guides/gender-equality-index-2021-report/gender-and-intersecting-inequalities-access-health?language_content_entity=en

Page 235 From what I see, and, sadly, this is backed by global stats, you're either in a low-paid, female-dominated profession or in a profession in which you're lower paid than men.
International Labour Organization (Feb. 2022). The gender gap in employment: What's holding women back? InfoStories. Retrieved from https://www.ilo.org/infostories/en-GB/Stories/Employment/barriers-women#intro.

Page 237 Music is a great comfort in palliative care.
Cavalli-Price, J. (2 Dec. 2020). The soothing role of music in hospice care. Music in Hospices. Retrieved from https://www.musicinhospices.org.uk/post/the-soothing-role-of-music-in-hospice-care.

WOMEN ARE ANGRY

Page 237 She talked about how gently humming soothed and centred her, how the comforting vibrations filled the inside of her body and kept external aggravations out.

Room 217 (2020). Guide for using music in hospice palliative care: Music collections and more. Retrieved from https://irp.cdn-website.com/6f97673f/files/uploaded/Guide%20for%20Using%20Music%20in%20HPC%20FINAL.pdf.

Page 237 Suzette would get through entire Nina Simone records without most people noticing.

Gallagher, L. M., Lagman, R., & Rybicki, L. (2018). Outcomes of music therapy interventions on symptom management in palliative medicine patients. *American Journal of Hospice and Palliative Care*, *35*(2), 250–7.

Page 242 That legacy seems to steer us, as we move through our professional lives and beyond.

Germano, M. (27 Mar. 2019). Women are working more than ever, but they still take on most household responsibilities. *Forbes*. Retrieved from https://www.forbes.com/sites/maggiegermano/2019/03/27/women-are-working-more-than-ever-but-they-still-take-on-most-household-responsibilities/?sh=6f34a02852e9.

Page 244 The trouble with this is: our brains don't like it.

Sullivan, R. M. (2012). The neurobiology of attachment to nurturing and abusive caregivers. *The Hastings Law Journal*, *63*(6), 1553–70.

Page 244 I've had plenty of patients across the years who've implemented strategic separations – everything from formal annual handshakes to full-blown estrangement.

Coleman, J. (10 Jan. 2021). A shift in American family values is fueling estrangement. *The Atlantic*. Retrieved from https://www.theatlantic.com/family/archive/2021/01/why-parents-and-kids-get-estranged/617612/.

Page 248 This isn't a manifesto for reuniting families – absolutely not; a lot of them are just hopelessly lost and toxic – but it *is* a reminder to not throw parts of ourselves or experiences we aren't comfortable with back into the gap between us and other people, where they tend to fester.

Scharp, K. M., Thomas, L. J., & Paxman, C. G. (2015). 'It was the straw that broke the camel's back': Exploring the distancing processes communicatively constructed in parent–child estrangement backstories. *Journal of Family Communication*, *15*(4), 330–48.

ENDNOTES

Chapter Twelve: Get It All Out

Page 255 In order to help this apparatus best inform our lives, we want to operate within a state of calm and conservation, where energy is spent on 'resting and digesting', as opposed to states in which the sympathetic 'fight or flight' system dominates.
Tindle, J., & Tadi, P. (2022). Neuroanatomy, parasympathetic nervous system. *StatPearls* [internet]. Retrieved from https://www.ncbi.nlm.nih.gov/books/NBK553141/.

Page 255 The more time we spend in calmer states, the more our bodies are allowed to get on with their own regulation, and the complexities of homeostasis (the stable conditions needed for survival).
Porges, S. W. (2022). Polyvagal theory: A science of safety. *Frontiers in Integrative Neuroscience, 16*, 871227.

Page 255 Persistent time spent in such sympathetic arousal states means our bodies are forced to contend with raised levels of cortisol and adrenaline, which over time, can do real damage.
Office on Women's Health (17 Feb. 2021). Stress and your health. Retrieved from https://www.womenshealth.gov/mental-health/good-mental-health/stress-and-your-health.

Page 256 As you're coming into consciousness, kick things off with a really good stretch to get your blood flow going and gently wake up your muscles.
Sudo, M., & Ando, S. (2020). Effects of acute stretching on cognitive function and mood states of physically inactive young adults. *Perceptual and Motor Skills, 127*(1), 142–53.

Page 256 Stretching is great for increasing positive emotion, encouraging dynamic interplay between brain activity and the nervous system.
Imagawa, N., Mizuno, Y., Nakata, I., Komoto, N., Sakebayashi, H., Shigetoh, H., ... & Miyazaki, J. (2023). The impact of stretching intensities on neural and autonomic responses: Implications for relaxation. *Sensors, 23*(15), 6890.

Page 256 Breathe like a baby, from your stomach: you're a primitive being, you're a mammal-baby again. Occupy *this* body on waking.
Hamasaki, H. (2020). Effects of diaphragmatic breathing on health: A narrative review. *Medicines, 7*(10), 65.

Page 257 As you enter into the day, attempt hourly body scans.
Gibson, J. (2019). Mindfulness, interoception, and the body: A contemporary perspective. *Frontiers in Psychology, 10*, 475917.

Page 257 Our brain and proprioception (our sense of our body in space) is all mapped through bodily receptors, signifiers which are entirely sensory.

Pathways.org (2023). What is proprioception? Understanding the 'body awareness' sense. Retrieved from https://pathways.org/what-is-the-proprioception-sense/.

Page 263 This is the road to assertiveness.
Gazipura, A. (2017). *Not Nice*. B. C. Allen Publishing.

Page 263 This is the road to standing our ground.
Reid, R. (2022). *The Power of Rude*. Trapeze.

Page 267 There are a hundred fast hacks for this online: alternate nostril breathing, pressure points, visualisations.
Mind (2024). Relaxing and calming exercises. Retrieved from https://www.mind.org.uk/need-urgent-help/what-can-i-do-to-help-myself-cope/relaxing-and-calming-exercises/.

Page 268 We're trying to ward off envious attack.
Flake Matsoso, A. (8 Aug. 2022) Envy, the wall between women. *Public Square Magazine*. Retrieved from https://publicsquaremag.org/dialogue/tolerance/envy-the-wall-between-women/.

Page 270 We're scared we'll be killed if we push it or assert a need, so better keep the peace.
Women's Aid (2024). Why don't women leave abusive relationships? Retrieved from https://www.womensaid.org.uk/information-support/what-is-domestic-abuse/women-leave/.

Page 271 It's of note that, these days, corporate buzz-speak clusters around 'using vulnerability' in decision-making.
Schmidt, L. (n.d.). Vulnerability in the workplace: A leadership skill. World of Work Project. Retrieved from https://worldofwork.io/2020/01/vulnerability-in-the-workplace/.

ENDNOTES

Page 271 As women, we're used to being trapped inside other people's projections and demands.
Nejatian, M., Alami, A., Momeniyan, V., Delshad Noghabi, A., & Jafari, A. (2021). Investigating the status of marital burnout and related factors in married women referred to health centers. *BMC Women's Health*, *21*(25).

Page 271 From our earliest family attachments, we're conditioned to react and respond to cues to perform along certain lines of expectation.
Hurry, A., Novick, J., & Novick, K. K. (1976). Freud's concept of projection. *Journal of Child Psychotherapy*, *4*(2), 75–88.

Page 272 What we're talking about here is the reality that, as a woman, you're probably far more likely to be worrying about telling someone how *you* feel and worrying that *you* must be the one in the wrong, that your very thoughts and feelings are the wrong things.
Kay, K., & Shipman, C. (May 2014). The confidence gap. *The Atlantic*. Retrieved from https://www.theatlantic.com/magazine/archive/2014/05/the-confidence-gap/359815/.

Page 272 The very fabric on which every institution and idea is built is predicated on the idea of men's superiority and power.
Ananthaswamy, A., & Douglas, K. (18 Apr. 2018). The origins of sexism: How men came to rule 12,000 years ago. *New Scientist*. Retrieved from https://www.newscientist.com/article/mg23831740-400-the-origins-of-sexism-how-men-came-to-rule-12000-years-ago/.

Page 273 There are some things we simply can't control.
Prasko, J., Ociskova, M., Vanek, J., Burkauskas, J., Slepecky, M., Bite, I., ... & Juskiene, A. (2022). Managing transference and countertransference in cognitive behavioral supervision: Theoretical framework and clinical application. *Psychology Research and Behavior Management*, *15*, 2129–55.

Final Note: What Now?

Page 280 Or: 'Addressing the global 75 per cent who are carers ...'
Barnes, S. B., & Ramanarayanan, D. (Apr. 2022). Global health & gender policy brief, no. 1. Wilson Center. Retrieved from https://www.wilsoncenter.org/sites/default/files/media/uploads/documents/The%20Care%20Economy%20-%20MHI%20Policy%20Brief%20Apr%202022.pdf.

WOMEN ARE <u>ANGRY</u>

Page 280 Or: '64 million jobs were lost due to the COVID-19 pandemic! Translating to $800 billion dollars' worth of income!'
International Labour Organization (25 Jan. 2021). ILO monitor: COVID-19 and the world of work. 7th edition. Retrieved from https://www.ilo.org/global/topics/coronavirus/impacts-and-responses/WCMS_767028/lang--en/index.htm.

Page 281 We aren't modelling something moderate and 'good enough', in the words of the paediatrician-psychoanalyst Donald Winnicott.
Winnicott, D. W. (1973). *The Child, the Family, and the Outside World.* Penguin, 173.

Page 283 As have the reasons for the dominant rates of major depression in women.
Zhao, L., Han, G., Zhao, Y., Jin, Y., Ge, T., Yang, W., ... & Li, B. (2020). Gender differences in depression: Evidence from genetics. *Frontiers in Genetics, 11.*